Coconut Head's
Cancer Survival Guide
My Journey from Diagnosis to "I Do"

HOLLY J. BERTONE

DEDICATION

To my Warrior Sisters.   May you find peace, support, inspiration, beauty, and happiness.

ACKNOWLEDGEMENTS

To God for his blessings in disguise.

To my boys (Carter and Stepson) for standing by my side every step of the way and for their unconditional love.

To my parents for teaching me about fortitude, which helped me get through this.

To my doctors and medical team for providing the best treatment and saving my life.

To my family and friends for standing by me through breast cancer, and their encouragement to share my story.

To my editor, Emily Yee, and my graphic artist, Jenn at Munchkin Land Designs for their final touches on making this book a reality.

INTRODUCTION

This whole project started as something simple – a few emails to 10 of my closest family and friends to let them know I had been diagnosed with breast cancer and keep them posted on my condition and progress. The email chain grew in numbers, and writing became my therapy. Despite wanting to keep my struggles "private," many folks found these emails inspiring and suggested I should turn them into a blog, and eventually a book. So I did.

I filled in the blanks and made very few edits. I wanted to keep it raw, so you the reader can experience where I was before, during, and after treatment. That being said, please lower your expectations on literary excellence, as Hemingway I am not. But if I can inspire just one person with this book, then it's all worth it to take a very private struggle public.

Everyone responds to cancer differently. When I was diagnosed, I didn't have a choice to have cancer, but I did have a choice as to how to respond. You can be depressed about it, or you can laugh through it. I chose to laugh through it. Fortunately, my husband shared the same sentiment. By no means is any of the humor in this book meant to be disrespectful of cancer patients or survivors in any way. Humor was simply our way of coping and laughing through a very difficult and painful year of our lives.

To the cancer patients and survivors – Whatever you are feeling or whatever you are going through, it's normal. You can do this. You are beautiful. You are strong. I have faith in you.

To the caretakers (family and friends) – I know the only thing you want to do is take away the cancer and make your loved one whole again. You can't. Just be there, listen to your loved one, and respond to their needs.

Regardless of who you are reading this book, I hope you find your own inspiration and realize you are not alone. Use this opportunity to evaluate your life and make some positive changes. On the days you feel the lowest, find something small to do, something that gives you reason to hold your head high and be proud of you.

Love and hugs from your Warrior Sister,

Holly

LIFE AT FIVE YEARS OUT

I can't believe how fast five years has come and gone. It's like I blinked and went from cancer diagnosis to celebrating my five-year survivorversary. Of course, while going through everything, it felt like the end of the world. But now it's a distant memory. Crystal clear yet blurry. Life altering. A place I would never want to go back to, but a place I'm extremely glad I came from.

To celebrate five years, I am re-releasing *The Coconut Head's Cancer Survival Guide* and sharing my top five life-balancing mantras that I learned in the last five years since diagnosis.

Know Your Priorities

My health actually declined after treatment ended. I was more sick after treatment than I was during treatment. I was in recovery and still struggling. When my boss said to me, "Your health and your family don't matter," I knew I had to make a change. Immediately.

I had spent the first 20 years of my career climbing the corporate ladder with enormous success. At this point, I didn't have to prove anything to anyone. My health and family absolutely do matter. They are worth more than any job or income. I walked away from one of the highest positions in the Federal government without any regrets. I now work a normal job with normal hours. I have zero stress at work, and I'm home in time to care for Stepson after school. My health and my family matter more than anything. Period. Nothing will get in the way of either one.

Know Your Fortitude

It took my doctors an entire year after treatment ended to figure out what was wrong with me. I was diagnosed with Hashimoto's, which is a thyroid disease. My guess is that chemo and/or radiation knocked my thyroid out of whack, but we will never know for certain the actual cause. Despite the diagnosis and subsequent medicine, I still felt sick. I struggled with extreme fatigue, migraines, stomach aches, space shuttle launches in the bathroom five to six times a day, dizziness... the list goes on. Between chemo and Hashi's, I thought that feeling this way was my lot in life. I thought that I would have to struggle every day for the rest of my life, so I did what I could to survive and only complained when it got really bad. I was confident in my choice for treatment and accepted having to feel this way was the smaller price to pay to do away with the chance of cancer coming back.

Every day, I woke up sick and did a mental self check, "Do I feel better or worse than I did during cancer?" And then went about my day pretending that my health was normal. Compared to cancer, pretty much everything else that life hands you is the equivalent to a hangnail. I told myself day in and day out, "If I can get through cancer, I can make it through today."

In weakness comes strength.

Know Your Body

In February 2015, six months shy of my five-year survivorversary, I had a light bulb moment. I conducted my own research like my life depended on it. Because it did. I learned that my "healthy eating" was actually what was harming me. Due to the chemo and Hashi's, some prolific inflammation kicked in and set my auto-immune system on overdrive. I was eating the correct nutrients, but my body was rejecting them. Toxins were leaking into my bloodstream and causing my body to attack itself.

Overnight and completely cold turkey I went 100% gluten free and then became a "pesco-baco vegan." Within three weeks, the fatigue was manageable, and the stomach aches and migraines were gone. And in case you are concerned about my BMs - totally normal! I eliminated additional foods on the Autoimmune Protocol such as corn, nightshades, peanuts, and quinoa. A food sensitivity blood panel came back to confirm what I had already put into action. It wasn't the chemo or the Hashis which was causing me to be sick every day, it was my food. Within four months, I was about 90% back to my old self. I felt "normal" and started back into an exercise program. After four and a half years, I was able to begin enjoying life again the way it should be enjoyed.

My story and my journey are extreme, but I am so completely blessed to have been able to listen to my body and push for answers. I've used my blog as an awareness platform to tell my story, because whether it's cancer, thyroid issues, food issues, or anything else... too often as women we are scared to rock the boat. We take care of everyone else, but we don't take care of ourselves. I urge you to listen to your body and don't be afraid to keep pushing for answers when you feel that something is wrong.

Know Your Passion and Purpose

Throughout this journey, I've become completely focused on my mission and purpose in life. As of this writing, I still work full time outside of the home but am making progress every day to walk away for good. My blog has given me the opportunity to connect with and inspire so many women. I've changed the focus to be more home and family based with articles on decor, design, DIY, recipes, family, inspiration, healthy living, etc but it's still a platform for me to share my story and raise awareness for early detection of cancer.

In addition to this book, I've written an e-book called *Drops of Fortitude* which is a short e-read. I also published a children's book *My Mommy Has Cancer*. Each publication is an emotional experience, but I broke down when I received the children's book back from the publisher. It was written from a child's perspective to talk to another child about cancer and is illustrated by children of survivors. It was published last year on my four-year survivorversary.

Earlier this year, Hubby and I realized our dream of opening an eBay store. I thought blogging was fun, but I am out of my mind excited to work the store. We both have a passion for hitting up yard sales, flea markets, thrift stores, and antique stores and are always on the lookout for fun and unique items to sell on the store.

There is a level of peace that comes with being in the place you know you are supposed to be and following your passion and purpose in life. I am living my life with no regrets.

Know Your True Beauty

Going through cancer treatment will deliver an epic blow to the ole self esteem. Recovery is difficult both physically and emotionally. The inner scars are typically deeper than the external ones.

This one has been stirring inside of me for a while. I knew that there was a missing piece to my purpose and passion, but I wasn't sure what it was. Like everything else in life, it just kind of happened. I knew that the last piece of the puzzle was to find beauty in the broken.

I created a special collection on our eBay store to sell upcycled and repurposed creations. These items parallel my journey as a breast cancer survivor, and the journey to find true beauty. Each item in the store is one-of-a-kind and handmade (by yours truly). They are pieces that were old, and/or rusted, and/or covered in dirt and cobwebs, and/or ready for the trash or landfill. They are the pieces that everyone else thinks are worthless and should be thrown away. With a little bit of creativity and a lot of love, I have resurrected these items into beautiful treasures. It's a way to honor real beauty and remind women to love yourself no matter what you are going through.

It's also a way for me to help fund my advocacy efforts. 100% of the profits from these sales will be channeled into Pink Fortitude, LLC's breast cancer awareness and advocacy program via book donations to cancer centers, awareness materials, and donations to The Tigerlilly Foundation and The Dr. Susan Love Research Foundation.

A cancer diagnosis is like being hit with a ton of bricks. It feels like there is no light at the end of the tunnel. But let me encourage you, my friend, to look beyond today. Whether you have been given a "good" diagnosis or are at Stage IV and/or terminal, your life has purpose. You may be sick, but every single day you have a choice as to how you are going to live your life. You can be a victim and wallow in the woe is me, or you can make a difference and inspire others.

As you read this book and my story, I challenge you to look beyond today. There will be times to cry, there will be times to laugh. But most importantly, there will be a time to define or re-define who you are.

Let me know how you are doing - I would love to connect with you! Please follow me on social media @PinkFortitude and drop me a line at holly@coconutheadsurvivalguide.com to say hello.

FORWARD FROM MY HUSBAND, CARTER

Holly and I met the old-fashioned way. We met in a bar.

I was drunk, having a bad day, and getting my beer on after work with some co-workers. Holly was sitting by herself, clearly waiting for a friend. I have a rule – I always talk to a good looking red head. And there she was.

I summoned some liquid courage, swaggered up to her, and asked if I could sit next to her.

"I'm waiting for my friend," Holly said abruptly, wanting nothing to do with me.

"Well then, I will just sit here until your friend shows up," I replied. I tried to make small talk. The more I tried, the more it was clear I was getting nowhere fast. They said when you find yourself in a hole, quit digging. So in a desperate last-ditch effort to advance conversation with this beautiful woman, I threw a Hail Mary.

"You know," I said, "there are two kinds of people in this world – Stones people and Beatles people. Which one are you?"

"Beatles," she replied, as if it was the only choice.

"Well, it's clear there is no future in this relationship," I turned my back on her.

She tapped my shoulder, "but why?"

TOUCHDOWN! That line always works. The rest they say is history, and this Stones guy fell head over heels for the Beatles girl.

Little did I know, the same carefree girl who sang KC and the Sunshine Band off key yet at the top of her lungs on the night we met would be the same woman who would fight for her life to beat breast cancer. Little did I know, the same girl with long curly red hair who I had to chat up at the bar that night would be sick and bald on our wedding day.

This is her story. This is our story.

LIFE BEFORE CANCER
Friday, July 30, 2010

My life was perfect. I was 18 days away from my 39th birthday. I was living with my boyfriend Carter and his son aka "Stepson". For the last few months, Carter had started introducing me as his fiancé, and we were looking at rings. In five days, we would be heading up to see his family in upstate New York, and I was sure he was going to propose before we went or while we were there so his mother could see the ring.

For the last 10 years of being single in my thirties, I had bought a home, I dated a lot, I got my master's degree, I climbed the corporate ladder, I traveled to fabulous places, I raced my mountain bike and XTerras, I rock climbed, I drank margaritas with my girlfriends. I had a carefree life where I could pick up and do anything at any time. I was happy.

When Carter and I met, I wasn't ready to give up my single life. But over time, he won me over, and I knew I was ready to commit to being his wife and a stepmother to his son. I did everything I had ever wanted to do as a single gal, and I was ready to settle down with no regrets. I was ready to change my focus from having fun and doing my own thing, to taking care of my new family. I was excited for this time in my life and excited for a new beginning.

THE TORNADO AND A RED KATE SPADE BAG
Saturday, July 31, 2010

I woke up and felt a small lump on the right side of my right breast. "Carter... I don't think this should be here. Is this normal? Should this be here?" Carter gave sage advice to call my doctor first thing Monday morning because regardless of whether it was something or nothing, I would worry about it.

Monday, August 2, 2010

8:01am. I called my primary doctor's office and explained I had found a lump.

2:00pm. I was sitting on the exam table and fortunately, my primary doctor "Dr. R." the doctor who I've had for the last 10 years and is the best primary doctor in the world, made room in her schedule to see me. Trying to strike the balance of being judicious but not worrying, she told me that lumps like this are normal and women my age (pre-40) are typically lumpy and bumpy, but she wrote a script for a mammogram and told me to call right away.

2:30pm. In the parking lot of the doctor's office. I called the lab to see if they could still see me that day. Unfortunately they could not.

Wednesday, August 4, 2010

I had my first mammogram. Now, for those of you not in the know... it's not like a TSA agent being able to see a bright white outline of your hairdryer as your luggage passes through the X-ray screener. There is no clear, defined object. The lab tech analyzes gray shadows. "Look, here's your lump." I thought of the Friends episode where

3

Rachel was getting an ultrasound and felt like a bad mother because she couldn't see her baby on the screen. All I could see were shades of gray. That night, when Carter asked how it was, I responded, "Imagine your junk being slammed in the refrigerator door." The conversation was dropped.

The worst part of this experience was that I had some shoulder pain recurrence from an old mountain bike injury and was taking ibuprofen. They gave me the results immediately. I needed a biopsy, but because I was taking ibuprofen, they would not do it that day and I had to wait a week. They didn't tell me I had cancer, but I knew. I knew at that very moment that I had cancer. The pit in your stomach doesn't lie. The following morning, Carter, Stepson, and I had plans to drive up to upstate NY for a few days of vacation time at his parent's house in the mountains. It weighed heavy the entire time.

Friday, August 13, 2010

It was Friday the 13th. Carter drove me to the biopsy, which was a smart move to make. The procedure was a lot more painful and invasive than I had anticipated. After the biopsy, they took me in for another mammogram, during which I was so woozy from the procedure, I came very close to passing out. The nurse gave me some smelling salts. Carter drove me home and I slept the remainder of the day.

Saturday, August 14, 2010

Carter was out of town for the weekend. Facing the possibility of having breast cancer, I did what any rational female would do... RETAIL THERAPY, baby! I was still in some pain, but I needed to get out and occupy my time. I ended up at the Kate Spade outlet. My reasoning was, I needed a "mom bag"... bigger and more durable than my purse to carry things like baseball gloves and DS games. In reality, I knew in the back of my mind, I would be in for a lot of doctors appointments and wanted a separate bag for the journey. I ended up with a red bag. Because if you gotta have cancer, you may as well also have a most fabulous red Kate Spade bag.

THE CALL
Wednesday, August 18, 2010

JFK. Challenger. 9/11. Poignant moments that transcend time... they remain so vivid you could ask anyone where they were that day, what they were doing, even what they were wearing, and the details would be recalled with immaculate precision.

I met up with Carter to commute home together on the Metro. We jumped on the Blue Line train. I had an outside seat beside a woman, and he stood about four rows in front of me. In a typical DC rush hour on a sweltering August day, the train was hot and packed and standing room only. Between the Reagan Airport and Braddock Road stops, my phone rang. It was my primary doctor's office. Another doctor was on the phone and calling because Dr. R. was on vacation and out of town. A packed train isn't quiet. I strained to hear the doctor, and I'm sure was shouting my responses in the crowd.

"I'm calling with your test results. I'm sorry to let you know... you have breast cancer." He then said something like, "fortunately, it's the good kind" and then went into medical-ese to give me the clinical details of my tumor...invasive ductal carcinoma. Ummm.... there's a good kind of breast cancer? Huh? He went on to discuss next steps, which included finding a good surgeon because I would need to have a lumpectomy to remove the tumor.

"That's a silly name for such an important surgery," I replied. Odd, yes, but how else was I supposed to respond? I wrote down all of the information he gave me and hung up. I looked up for Carter. It was another stop before I could connect with him and let him know.

Google was my best friend and worst enemy that night. And invasive ductal carcinoma didn't sound very good.

Note #1 – A week or so later, I received the paperwork in the mail. It was dated August 17. So while I received the phone call the day after my birthday, I technically received the diagnosis on my birthday. Months later, I would make the decision to make August 17th my Survivorversary.

Note #2 - There is no perfect way to break the news, "you have cancer." I appreciated the phone call, because after waiting 18 days after initially finding the lump, I didn't want to wait another day or two or more to go into my doctor's office just for them to break the news and then have to wait another few days to schedule another appointment with another doctor who could treat me from that point on. Despite the surroundings, I'm glad I got the call over the phone rather than waiting for an appointment. And I actually felt bad for that doctor who had to step in and make such a life-altering phone call to a patient he had never met.

Note #3 - After being thrown knee deep into it, I found out there are a gazillion types of breast cancer depending on the markers and combinations. I certainly wouldn't call one good or bad, as all cancer is bad... but there are many variations of tumor size and aggressiveness that will impact treatment type and length. Most women who get breast cancer are over the age of 55. For the women who get breast cancer under the age of 40, it is typically an aggressive kind. Fortunately, mine was lazy ("clinical" description from my surgeon).

48 HOURS. 8 MAGIC WORDS
Friday, August 20, 2010

Carter got down on one knee with the most beautiful ring and proposed. It was the moment most girls dream of. And it was. In 48 hours, my life was turned upside down by eight magic words, "You have breast cancer," and "Will you marry me." It was extra poignant because not only did he propose, but he still wanted to marry me even though I had breast cancer.

Now… here's where the fun begins. Because anyone not in the situation, would say, "Girlfriend, you are nuts! Of course he still wanted to marry you." But the minute the cancer thing hits, it takes over your brain and makes you think totally irrational things. Including lots of self-doubt. Stay tuned, because this whole self-doubt will get crazy as the weeks and months pass.

DIAGNOSIS

The first doctor I met with was Dr. S., a breast cancer surgeon. She was very matter of fact with the perfect side dose of empathy. I took lots of notes, but she also wrote everything down for me and drew diagrams of my surgery. While I never asked "why," I had secretly been wondering "how." Before I could even ask, she looked me straight in the eye and said, "You have a healthy lifestyle, you don't have any risk factors, and you don't have a family history of breast cancer. Lightning struck your breast." It's all I needed to know. I never asked why and I never asked how. All I wanted to do was fight it.

Dr. S. explained I was Estrogen/Progesterone (ER/PR) Positive, and HER-2 Negative. She explained, most women under 40 who have breast cancer get the aggressive kind. To use an official medical term, she called mine, "lazy." After she spent plenty of time explaining my diagnosis and treatment options, I did finally understand why the doctor who called with my diagnosis had said I had the good kind of cancer. We discussed the pros and cons of a lumpectomy over a mastectomy, and I actually got to be involved in the decision. I would have radiation after a lumpectomy. Chances were I would not need chemo, but if she were to find cancer in my lymph nodes, then chemo would be necessary.

I had decisions and a game plan.

OUR ENGAGEMENT

Most newly engaged couples pick out china patterns and decide honeymoon destinations. We decided my surgery would be at Virginia Hospital Center in Arlington. Most brides try on dresses and veils. I tried on wigs because I was going to be bald on my wedding day. Dinner conversations were not about whether the invitations should be white, cream, ivory, or ecru. Dinner conversations were about having a lumpectomy over a mastectomy. We talked about cancer. All. The. Time. Because we had to deal with it, and because there were a lot of decisions to make.

But we chose only to share the good news of the engagement, and not the bad news of the cancer. Simultaneously, Carter was retiring from the military after 25 years and looking for a job in the civilian world. It was too much to process, and we wanted to keep the cancer private for as long as we could. It was like we were living two completely separate lives. To the outside world, we were happy and newly engaged. Behind closed doors, every single conversation was filled with angst. The mood in the house was not lovey dovey as most engaged couples get to experience. The tension was so thick you could cut it with a knife.

We chose to not even tell my parents at first. My mother was scheduled for heart surgery in the upcoming weeks, and I didn't want the news to break her heart prematurely. So we waited.

Because my cancer was ER/PR positive, my surgeon told me to stop taking birth control pills immediately. I looked at her trying to hold back the tears and asked for a one week extension. We needed one week for something to be normal in our lives. I kept my promise and one week later, I stopped taking the pill. Forever.

Looking back, I think the first few weeks after diagnosis were the worst. Even harder than dealing with chemo. There was so much uncertainty. Our lives had crumbled in an instant. Nothing would ever be the same. Ever. It was devastating. It was too much to handle. And we didn't know where to turn. We talked. We cried. We bickered. But we figured it out.

CARTER'S TURN

Holly is as healthy as a horse, so I didn't think anything of it the morning she asked me to check the lump on the side of her breast. "It's probably nothing," I reassured her. "But you should have it looked at." I'm a better-safe-than-sorry kind of guy, and I always like to take care of things immediately. Well, except for maybe taking out the trash or hanging up blinds.

We were riding home on the Metro together when Holly received the call from the doctor's office. Her demeanor changed immediately. Something was definitely wrong, and I could tell she was trying to keep a "brave face."

The news was not good.

In that moment, everything changed, yet nothing changed.

I proposed two days later.

SURGERY
Wednesday, September 29, 2010

In typical guy fashion, all Carter wanted to do was fix me. He couldn't, and it made him mad that I had to go through this.

In the hospital when I was waiting for surgery, a women came in and explained she was there to hold my hand during a little procedure. She politely told Carter to go out and get some breakfast, it would be about 20 minutes before I came back. They rolled me down to another room, and this woman, this angel, held my hand. I realized why. The other nurse stuck a needle where needles should not go. Now mind you, this had all been explained by my doctor. But like everything else, it was blah blah blah blah CANCER blah blah blah blah. How I missed having a needle stuck THERE is beyond me. O.M.G. it hurt. The procedure was to inject dye so my surgeon could see if the cancer had spread to my lymph nodes. I kissed Carter and went into surgery.

I woke up and asked the nurse to tell Carter I was ok but needed a few minutes. The first thing I did was to wiggle my fingers and toes. My arm hurt.

Carter came in to see me. He had tears in his eyes. If I ever doubted his love for me, at that moment I knew for certain. He told me they had found small traces of cancer in the lymph nodes, and chemo was now on the table.

The artist formerly known as the tumor was removed, along with clear margins. It was 1.3 cm which is about the size of a thumbnail. There was still much uncertainty.

THE TURNING POINT
September 30, 2010

The day after surgery, I was flat on the couch in pain, because I didn't want to take the pain meds. We had already exhausted the TV and DVD collection, and Carter was sitting on the chair bored to tears.

"You up for some…..?" He looked over and asked me.

"Are you crazy?" I laughed.

"I'm bored."

I couldn't stop laughing. My betrothed is seriously deranged. And that was the turning point. We started laughing, and it was much needed.

From that point on, we could laugh at and with cancer. And it felt much better. Now, there were still plenty of moments for lots of tears, but it was easier to deal with cancer by laughing.

FOUNDATIONAL ISSUES

One thing I learned very early is that many, many brave women before me had sacrificed to pay it forward for my generation of treatment. I think it's just one of those things you do...you don't want anyone else to go through what you did... and you try to make it better for the next generation of women who have breast cancer. I didn't start writing my journal until I was knee deep into treatment. Let me go back in time and share with you a very ugly day at the beginning of treatment and a very ugly side of breast cancer. It was also the turning point when I decided that despite being a cancer patient, I was not going to be a cancer victim, and was not going to let cancer take everything away from me. I had to fight back. I had to take control.

Back in September, facing surgery, I was more concerned with losing my hair than dealing with having a lucky fin. I'm not buxomous, and I never even thought the partial mastectomy (aka lumpectomy) would bother me. Well, immediately after surgery, it did. Being newly engaged, I wanted to be a beautiful, sexy fiancé and bride. Carter's preference was that I be alive and healthy (and still told me I was sexy and beautiful - yep he's a keeper). Not only was it dealing with the scars and lucky fin, but nothing fit or felt good any more. I went to eight different stores with the same results - nothing fit, nothing felt good, and the selections were horrid (and the week after surgery, shopping for new bras was NOT fun). I ended up at Victoria's Secret. And in the middle of VS with nothing fitting right or feeling good (AGAIN)... cue the meltdown of epic proportion. I'm talking hysterics and big crocodile tears. I drove straight home, ran upstairs, and slammed the bedroom door. Carter came up immediately to console me and had me laughing within minutes.

After the meltdown subsided, I wrote a letter to Victoria's Secret. Now, it took me a few months and a few friends (THANK YOU!!!) to finish it and send it. But I did. I told my story and outlined a few small modifications they can do to one of their lines to make their foundational garments more comfortable for women going through breast cancer surgery and treatment. And for a company that donates A LOT of money to breast cancer through their parent organization, and considering they sell foundational garments (hello) I thought it would be a perfect fit for them not just modify one of their lines, but also use this as breast cancer awareness (hello October campaign!).

Well, I wrote the letter because it was the right thing to do, and I needed to take control of cancer. And it was another great turning point for me. I never wanted to feel like that again and I needed to show cancer who was boss. I needed to take back some control over the whole situation. I also knew that something good was going to happen. I didn't know what. But I knew I had cancer for a reason, and it was God's plan for me to turn it into something positive. I was excited about the unknown open doors and opportunities this would bring. I was excited to do something, but I had no idea what it would be. I knew something was burning inside.

Honestly... I thought it would go into a black hole...and totally forgot about it. But I received correspondence that they received the letter, and they were "taking my recommendations very seriously." Of course it was a form letter, and of course I still think it's in a black hole. Who knows if anything will come to fruition. But I tried my best to do one thing to make a difference for the next generation of women dealing with breast cancer.

[I ended up at Nordies, because they do a custom fitting, and had a sales woman dedicated to helping breast cancer patients.]

MAGIC 8 BALL

I've never had so many tests in my life. One was called an Oncotype DX. This test is not for everyone, but it's used to provide additional and personalized information in going forward with cancer treatment. It produced a super cool graph and chart of all of my markers. My three doctors reviewed the test and were back and forth as to the best standard of treatment. It was frustrating, because after surgery, I wanted to keep fighting and keep moving forward, and it took a couple weeks for my doctors to agree on next steps. Dr. D. explained the results, and I ended up right in the middle. It did not clearly show if chemo would actually work.

I'm sitting in her office. Holding a piece of paper, which was supposed to tell me what to do. And it didn't. I was completely helpless, and so was she.

"Ohhhh magic eight ball," I said shaking my hands together, "Should Holly get chemo or not?" Fortunately, Dr. D. has a sense of humor and chuckled at my attempt to lighten the situation.

"Right now, without chemo," she explained, "you have a 12% chance of recurrence. While we can't be 100% positive, based on your score, chemo would only reduce it to a 10% chance of recurrence."

"Let's go for it," I replied. "I'm a 10% kinda gal."

"Me too." She had me at hello.

CHEMO 101
Wednesday, November 3, 2010

Before chemo started, I took a two-hour prep course at the hospital. Just like the SAT prep course, they were thorough and prepared all of us for the big test ahead. They went through the different drugs we would be injected with, how it would work, various side effects, what we could and couldn't do in the infusion room, etc. All in all, it was a great class and worth the time to ease some of the worries of what chemo would be like.

But there were several aspects that were not discussed. Ever really wondered what it's like?

1. Chemo coursing through your body feels like a bad case of the flu. It's as simple as that. And although chemo affects everyone differently, this is the best way to describe it. You may or may not throw up, but the overall feeling is like having the flu and being achy and not wanting to do or able to do anything except sleep or lay on the couch.

2. You will smell. Bad. Chemicals oozing out of your pores is probably one of the worst smells known to man. My pee smelled so bad I almost threw up. One night, when we were in bed, Carter not only commented about how bad I smelled, but rolled over to the other side of the bed so he didn't have to sleep near me. Nothing says beautiful sexy fiancé like smelling like chemofunk. A couple months after chemo ended, as my finger nails were starting to grow back, I decided to bite/rip the dead nail off to give the healthy nail room to grow. As I bit the nail off with my teeth, the most wretched smell came out of my finger nail. Even months after the fact, chemofunk was still in my body, and it is a smell I will never forget.

3.   You will have BM issues. Best to ask your doctor or nurse about this one as it can go either way based on the drugs you are given. Thank goodness, my infusion nurse gave me a little helpful hint as she whispered, "stool softener." My chemo drugs caused horrible, horrible constipation. Even with the stool softener, it was extremely painful to go to the bathroom. I cried during each BM after chemo. Nothing says beautiful sexy fiancé like screaming and crying through painful BMs.

4.   Your GI track goes haywire. And then some. Nothing says beautiful sexy fiancé like having the walking farts. All. The. Time. My Great Aunt Myrtle would be so proud.

There are 257 side affects you can experience from chemo. These were the unmentionables and some of my favorites. So yes… I was stinky and smelled like chemofunk, cried during each BM, and had the walking farts.

Why this man still wanted to marry me was beyond comprehension.

THE BEGINNING
November 7, 2010

{From here on, the majority of the book turns into a compilation of email and blog entries I sent to family and friends.}

Dear Family and Friends -

Most of you know by now but for the ones who don't, here is the quick update. The good news is that on 20 August, Carter proposed. We decided to focus on sharing the good news and keeping the bad news private for as long as we could. Two days prior, on 18 August, I received the phone call that after a month of numerous tests, I have breast cancer. No risk factors, no family history, and nothing in my DNA. Lightning hit (very technical medical term used by my surgeon). The tumor was small and completely removed on 29 September. It's still very rare for women under the age of 40 to get breast cancer (about 5% compared to diagnoses at later ages). Where most women who are young have the aggressive kind, fortunately, mine is lazy. The only time in my life where I've been happy with mediocrity.

I have a phenomenal team of doctors, nurses, and staff and after much deliberation, they decided on both chemo and radiation to make sure they zap anything that could potentially be hiding and help reduce my risk of recurrence. So that has been my life over the last four months. Oh yeah... and Carter retired from the military and he's on leave until the end of the year and has been looking for a new job and I got a big promotion at work. We seem to be collecting major life events like some people collect stamps or coins.

Chemo begins this week. I am beyond ready to get this started and over with. I spent the entire weekend running errands and prepping the house for DEFCON 1. I have all of the medicine and medical comforts ready, in addition to some very "chemo chic" hats and scarves and a fabulous wig and of course a ton of books and magazines and movies and a freezer full of food. Tonight Carter is taking me out for one last date night before I start looking like and feeling like a hot mess. I am getting my hair cut ahead of when it's supposed to fall out so I can donate it to Locks of Love. I took a two-hour chemo prep course to learn about what is to be expected, and while life will certainly be rough for the next few months, it really sounds very manageable (she says now). And considering how stressful work has been the last couple weeks, I'm actually at the point where I'm looking forward to chemo since I'll be home and able to rest LOL!!! Carter has been a huge support, and it's been such a blessing that he's been home to help out. And Stepson is very excited to see my bald head.

I very much appreciate all of the emails and cards and calls and prayers and good wishes and everyone checking up on me. Please don't be sad for me. Good things happen to good people and this is God's special gift to me. I'm happy. I'm healthy. And something very wonderful will happen because of this.

And so the journey continues.

Love and hugs,

Holly

CHEMICALS BETWEEN US
November 11, 2010

The night before chemo #1, I got three hours of sleep worrying about all the what-ifs and unknowns and started my day with a little bit of woe is me. I walked into the injection room to a young woman my age asking for the barf bucket and some ginger ale. She fortunately managed to keep everything down and we had a nice chat throughout our treatments. Her name is Anita, her husband Michael, and their two kids Lily, 7, and Peter, 5. Anita has Stage 4 terminal colon cancer that has spread to her bones. She doesn't have long to live and she is in constant pain. Our treatment schedules are different so I don't know if I'll ever see her again. But I will never forget her.

Holly: "How do you stay so positive knowing that this is terminal?"

Anita: "My goal is to create very special memories for my children and family every single day I'm still here."

Pause a moment for some reflection on that one.

If you have an extra minute or two, please keep Anita and her family in your prayers. As I was finishing up my treatment, an older husband and wife came in for joint chemo treatment. They both got hit at the same time... she has an aggressive breast cancer and he has lymphoma. While battling my own breast cancer has been certainly tough enough on me and my family, yesterday certainly put this into perspective as I am beyond blessed to be on the "easy" side of the cancer street. The treatment room itself is very nice. They have big comfy lounge chairs for us and the oncology nurses (aka drug dealers) are absolute angels. In addition to making new friends, I watched Breakfast at Tiffany's and read a little and ate a snack.

Today, I still felt fine and dandy for most of the day (hello steroids!). I went for a three-mile run around the lake here at home this morning. Then off to donate my hair. Melissa worked her magic cutting my hair to donate to Locks of Love, and also preserve my dignity through the process (I had her turn me around - I couldn't watch). It's a short Emma Watson type pixie cut until it falls out. Both Carter and Stepson approve and like the new style, but I'm still getting used to it. I sported a pink wig all day to keep it fun, and I haven't cried over the loss of my hair (yet). Then back to the hospital for my superman shot to help keep my white blood cells strong and healthy. I've been feeling a little tired and "off" tonight, but that is to be expected considering I just had three hours of toxic chemicals going through my body.

The agenda for the remainder of the weekend is rest and relaxation.

Love and hugs,

Holly

RESPECT THE DRAINO
November 15, 2010

So I go into this whole process like... chemo schemo... how bad can it be, right? Wow. Chemo kicked me to the curb. And let me be perfectly clear. THIS SUCKS! I have a whole new respect for the effects of toxic chemicals surging through your body killing all fast growing cells both good and bad. Fortunately, it does cycle through and while even today, on Day #6 I'm still down for the count, each day I'm feeling a little bit better.

A shout out to my friend Linda and fellow warrior sister... she used the analogy that chemo is like throwing napalm on a forest to kill an ant hill. It's the most perfect analogy. And I can only chuckle thinking about the quote from Apocalypse Now... "I love the smell of napalm in the morning." Which is ironic, because I can't smell anything anymore!

I've heard going through something like this will give you a new perspective on life. I've also heard that whatever kind of person you were before cancer, it will only exemplify that. Whatever - it will manifest itself in due time. I summoned every ounce of energy I had on Sunday morning and made my weekly pilgrimage to the grocery store. It was an out of body experience. Like watching a movie of the world spinning around you. Each step forward was a struggle. I noticed the people around me. In their own little worlds. Getting their groceries. Healthy. And grumpy. Why are you sad? Why are you frowning? I wanted to smack them all upside the head.

I've always counted my blessings so maybe this experience will make it even more so. Or maybe my new mission in life is to help others recognize their own blessings to count. So do me a favor today and be thankful for something.

23

Lord, let this toxic draino unclog whatever gunk it needs to in my drain today.

Love and hugs,

Holly

BALD IS BALD
December 6, 2010

Going through Round #1 of chemo was an experience, and now I'm much better prepared. The three-week cycle is ideal, as it's the first half of the days dealing with the effects and then the last half feeling somewhat normal. I was able to go back to work and do some light jogging on the treadmill, all at a much slower pace.

Right on schedule, Thanksgiving Day, my hair started coming out in clumps. We were up at Carter's parents in upstate New York, so his mom got out the clippers and Stepson helped by cleaning it up as it was shaved off. When we got home, Carter took the razor to it. The cancer cliche is, "bald is beautiful." I think it's more like... bald is just bald. I was very sad to have it finally all go and I miss my red hair. But hair is not love or friendship or health. It's just hair. And it will grow back. And ice cream and DQ therapy has been helping me cope!

Round #2 was this past Wednesday. It was physically tougher, but mentally easier so I guess that counts as a break-even. I'm hoping to be back at work tomorrow and back on the treadmill later this week. Two down. Two to go.

Love and hugs,

Holly

I DISAGREE WITH THE HEADLINES
December 8, 2010

Elizabeth Edwards did not "lose" her battle to breast cancer. Her grace, her strength, and her courage is an inspiration to millions. I consider that a victory.

"And my heaven will be a big heaven. And I will walk through the front door." (Peter Gabriel)

Love and hugs,

Holly

BALD'S ENCORE
December 9, 2010

Top 10 Reasons Why it's God's Plan to Lose Your Hair When You Go Through Chemo:

10. The money market fund I have to pay for curly hair styling products is now directed to chemo costs.

9. With "chemo brain," I would forget to turn off the curling iron and burn the house down.

8. If/when the hard core sickness happens... no worries about anyone having to hold my hair back while getting sick.

7. Fun new head accessories to wear.

6. One free wig compliments of insurance.

5. I'm now a good luck charm (must rub the bald head).

4. Keeps it in check - the trauma of losing my hair actually trumped the trauma of having cancer.

3. No more bad hair days - the worst it gets is the remaining stubble looking like a dog with mange, and that's pretty sexy.

2. More time to sleep in the morning - less time to get ready.

1. Not having to shave my legs (lost it there too) for the next several months is truly a very, very special gift from God.

Oh and as a bonus... and because it's so much fun to go there.... when else in life can you say, "Do these jeans make my head look bald!!!"

Love and Hugs,

Holly

MY 12 DAYS OF CHRISTMAS
December 19, 2010

The doctors tell you that the three-week chemo cycle is the best as you have the last 7 days or so at the end to feel "normal" before the next cycle begins. This time around, that was a bunch of hooey as I've been sick every day during my "7 days of normal." I'm sick of being sick. I remember one of the nurses warning me that most people are the worst going into their next-to-last treatment. But she cautioned... "I think it's mostly mental." Considering that I'm armed with a psychology degree, beating the mental is like acing a freshmen-level class. Mind over matter I just try to pretend that I feel ok and put one foot in front of the other. Plus, I have a very special Chemo Christmas to look forward to....

On the 12th day of Christmas my oncologist gave to me...

12 hours sleeping
11 crackers eating
10 G2 a drinking
9 scarves a wearing
8 steroids surging
7 Hoarders episodes a watching
6 drugs a dripping
5 days on the couch
4 infusion hours
3 days off work
2 infusion nurses
and one superman shot.

I'm going for a walk. Fake it til you make it.

Love, hugs, and good drugs, Holly

CH-CH-CH-CHANGES
December 21, 2010

All cancers have their challenges, and each one is unique. I've been very blessed that my side effects have been minor and manageable. And just when I think I have adjusted... but wait... there's more. Nothing says sexy fiancé like a young woman going through hot flashes. Or my eyes constantly watering and nose constantly running.

I honored my Great Aunt Myrtle with crumpled up tissues in my pockets to take care of my leaking face. That along with the walking farts and a couple of half eaten starlight mints attached to my sweater and I know she would be smiling in her grave. Ahhh... pause for happy memories.

And God bless Carter for being so supportive and such a good sport about all of the changes I've gone through over the last few months. His favorite way to keep us both laughing has been to come up with some funny nicknames, most of which are dedicated to my hair... er... or lack thereof. Here they are in order of disappearance:

1. Hank, my teenage son
2. Private Bertone
3. GI Jane
4. Sinead O'Connor
5. Dusty Cue Ball
6. Kojack
7. Pirate (argh)
8. Coconut Head
And of course Nemo, a shout out to my lucky fin.

To celebrate my body doubling in age, Carter is taking me out to Roy Rogers for dinner tonight... at 4:00 of course, so we are in home in time to watch Matlock and Murder She Wrote.

Love, hugs, and seven hours until more good drugs. Bring it.

Holly

MERRY CHEMO
December 22, 2010

Treatment #3 was yesterday, and according to the timing of my last treatments, I'll be down for the count for Christmas Eve and Christmas Day. My goal is to rally and make it to Christmas Eve service, regardless of how I feel (extra prayers welcome!). We shall see. Good intentions have sidelined me before with this.

My mother has threatened to call Pastor Sue to reserve the last pew with one of those big orange construction cones. That might be kind of tacky. But if it was decorated maybe like a Santa hat or Christmas tree, now that would be more than appropriate! I missed out on the standard December of baking and shopping and parties and being social, but it will be extra special to spend a quiet Christmas with Carter and my parents.

I don't know how my drug dealers (infusion nurses) can do this kind of work every day, but God bless them for it. The best news of all yesterday... and without getting into too many of the details... but my three doctors (and their colleagues around the country) were debating between four and six chemo treatments due to my case not being standard care (ohhhh magic 8-ball...). We were planning on four... with six always being out there. My oncologist confirmed four. It's in writing. Prayer answered. Go God!!!

I'm grateful to have such supportive family and friends, and thank you all for your prayers and cards and emails. It's great to know that I have Team Bertone behind me, especially on the days that are a little rougher than others, and your support really means a lot.

Count your blessings. Enjoy the holidays with your loved ones. Reflect on the memories of those not with us. Be nice to strangers. Spread joy. Hug more. May you and your family have a wonderful Christmas and holiday season.

Love, hugs, peace, and joy.

Holly

ALL THE WAY TO PARIS
December 26, 2010

It's really hard not to view this cancer thing as competition because I want to beat it every day and some days I just can't. I'm learning about the art of war in that sometimes you have to take a step back and understand that it's more important to strategize to win the entire war rather than each and every battle. Cancer was a buzz kill this Christmas. I was sick and slept a lot and never made it to Christmas Eve service. Cancer won some minor battles this weekend and that's ok. But I spent Christmas Eve and Christmas Day with the people who I love the most. And that is a much more important victory to me. Tiz the season for all of the hustle and bustle, and sometimes it's trying to find the quiet that feels the best.

"Let's have the guts to let the ba$tards go all the way to Paris. Then, we'll cut em off and chew em up." - General Patton/Seige of Bastogne (Christmas 1944).

Love, hugs, and strategizing for global domination.

Holly

ODE TO THE STUPID COUCH
December 28, 2010

Well the good news is that as bad as it hits... there is a rebound. I'm still recovering and not back to "normal," but I certainly feel much better. I am back at work and back to the gym and all is well in my world.

Thanks to surgery and chemo, it would only be fitting if I dedicated one of my musings to the Stupid Couch.

Ode to the Stupid Couch

When I am not feeling well
You comfort me for a spell
My bottom and you become one
Until my rest and healing is done
From too many episodes of Hoarders and What Not to Wear
At some point I just don't seem to care
When I don't have my get up and go
My IQ lowers with each show
I will always love you my dear Stupid Couch
And despite what Carter says, for you I will always vouch!

Love, hugs, and leaving a big imprint.

Holly

TWO ZERO ONE ONE
January 1, 2011

After close to two months of overindulgence, we pause as a people on 1 January to reflect on how we can be better. It's the same rhetoric of I want to: eat healthier, work out, connect more with family and friends, be a nicer person, volunteer more, save money, and leap tall buildings with a single bound. After the last two months of living the anti-overindulgence, I can't help but reflect on New Years past and the most important daily life decisions at the time:

1. Should I dump this guy before or after the second date?
2. How much air pressure should I have in my bike tires for the conditions on today's training ride?
3. What flavor of energy bar should I eat for dinner tonight?

My life was much simpler then.

2011 has some pretty big titles that I will be gaining. Wife. Stepmother. Cancer survivor. Do I still want to eat healthier, work out, connect more with family and friends, be a nicer person, volunteer more, save money and leap tall buildings with a single bound? Absolutely. But this year I'm not making any resolutions. All I want to do is get my health back to normal and take care of my boys.

And everything else will fall into place.

Love, hugs, and all the best for 2011.

Holly

A PRAYER FOR FRIDAY
January 2, 2011

One thing I learned very early is as much as you can plan with cancer... it has a mind of its own and an uncanny way of giving back the unexpected (both good and bad). That being said... I need one more very specific thing to happen before I can get excited about a count-down to my last chemo treatment. I need "good labs" on 7 January. The chemo kills all fast growing cells, both good and bad. The bad ones are supposed to die a very painful and gruesome death. But the good ones... these are the good cells that they keep super close tabs on to ensure that I'm healthy enough to go through each chemo treatment. The next five days are very critical. So I'm asking for some very specific prayers for good blood counts this week. Here's how it works...

1. White blood cells are my infection soldiers and most important blood counts. Thanks so far to post-treatment superman shots and me being slightly obsessive about being bubble girl and germ-free... my WBC groupings have been in the safe zone. My metric for chemo is to keep these counts high enough and stay out of the emergency room.

2. Red blood cells are my oxygen carriers. They have been consistently low and barely in the safe zone. Hence lots of tiredness and fatigue, and I'm out of breath often. The WBC grouping is of highest importance, but the RBC grouping is pretty significant too.

3. Platlets are my blood clotters and last and least on the list of indicators. So far, all very normal, and if I get a slight cut or knick I'm fine but these are the last indicators the doctors look at to clear me for next treatment.

When I go in for labs on Friday I hope to be cleared for my final treatment on 12 January... then the official count down can begin. Please pray for good blood counts this week. God will listen.

Love and hugs and good blood,

Holly

PAGING DICK CLARK
January 7, 2011

Thank you to each and every member of Team Bertone for your very specific prayers this week for my blood counts. My white blood cell grouping is where it should be. My red blood cell grouping is still low and progressively lower than the last check, but still (barely) in the safe zone. God very graciously answered your prayers and I'm clear for my last chemo treatment on 12 January.

It's great how everyone wishes me the best for my chemo days... but I keep saying those are the easy days. I get to sit in a super comfy recliner for three to four hours and have quiet time to watch movies or read magazines and come home and sleep and aside from being dizzy, woozy, and tired, all is well on treatment day. It's the next few days and weeks after when the rubber meets the road and the fight gets tough. My countdown is not for 12 January. My countdown is for 26 January. That is the final appointment when I see my oncologist and get final labs and she blesses me as "healthy" and free to be on my merry way and begin daily radiation treatment in February. My cancer treatments don't end after chemo... but it is a big milestone.

So please join me in a 19 day countdown to the end of chemo. There will be a disco ball dropping somewhere...

Love, hugs, and counting down to a rockin' 26 January eve. Party on. Excellent.

Holly

YENTA
January 9, 2011

I mentioned before about one of the more fun and exciting side effects of chemo is going through "The Change." And many thanks to my elder sisters in solidarity for your kind words of support. For some reason, every time I get a hot flash, I keep singing this song that I made up and I can't get it out of my head. It doesn't make the hot flash go away, but it makes me laugh. Quite the catchy tune...

To the chorus of "Match Maker" from Fiddler on the Roof.

Hot flashes, hot flashes
At least you're polite
You give me fair warning before you ignite.

Hot flashes, hot flashes
My face is all flushed
Don't need no makeup and don't need no blush.

Hot flashes, hot flashes
When it's 20 degrees
It's a day at the beach with a warm summer breeze.

Love, hugs, and sticking my bald coconut head in the freezer.

Holly

BRING IT
January 12, 2011

Go big or go home.

I remember a few years ago when I was taking Muay Thai (mixed martial arts/boxing)... I was paired with another gal for some sparring. As a Level I student, the instructor orchestrated all of our moves to practice, so we both knew the routine order of moves. My partner was executing offensive moves, and I was on defense. My blocks were successful, but then I missed a parry. The next thing I knew, there was a left hook attached to a pink glove... kapow... right in the kisser. I was stunned more than hurt. But let it be known that after being punched in the head, I amped up the level of focus and concentration and effort to make sure it never happened again. And it didn't. And it won't.

One last time. I'm ready. Hands wrapped. Gloves on. Bring it.

"And if you break my will... I will come back again... to destroy everything you stood for." LIVE.

Love, hugs, and two more toxic drugs.

Holly

EXPECT MIRACLES
January 13, 2011

Have I mentioned recently how wonderful my entire medical team is? Yesterday's final infusion included a special guest appearance from the wonderful and fabulous Kerstin.... armed with a new mantra for me as my graduation present: "Expect Miracles." Which of course had me thinking.... outside of the obvious... what exactly is a miracle? So I consulted several standard and random internet sources.

There is... Miracle on Ice, Miracle on 34th Street, Miracle Worker, Miracle of Birth, Miracle Mile, Miracle Bras, and Miracle Whip. None of which really apply... although I am kind of hungry for a sandwich. Moving on...

World English Dictionary - #2 "any amazing or wonderful event." And further down... "Where miracles are there certainly God is."

Random poster and most profound - "The miracle we hope for is not always the miracle we receive."

But here is what I find the most intriguing (Wiki). "A miracle is an unexpected event attributed to divine intervention."

If a miracle is an unexpected event, and we are to "Expect Miracles"... (If A=B, and B=C, then A=C)... then that means we are to expect the unexpected. Life in general has its ups and downs, its good days and bad, and its interesting turn of events. Life has an uncanny way of happening all around you regardless of whether you want it to or not, or whether you have cancer or not.

A good normal day is also a pretty good day with cancer. A bad normal day is an even worse day with cancer. And a bad cancer day...

well... those just suck. The other day was one of those days in that it was a bad normal day and then with a bad cancer day on top. (A secret to those who have lauded me for always being so positive - I sometimes manage to sneak in a few bad moments when no one is looking - kinda like that extra piece of chocolate. Shhhh - don't tell!). Some days the bigger miracles are needed, but most days it's the smaller ones. The simple ones that get you through the day and onto the next. The ones that you don't ask for but God knows you need.

This year already has a full plate for the soon-to-be Bertones, and it's only mid-January. So on top of donning the Supergirl cape and beating cancer, there's a lot of other big events going on in our lives. We need some wonderful events. It's time to expect the unexpected.

But right now it's time to grab the Glamour magazine and turn on the DVR recorded episodes of Hoarders and settle into the next four days of peace and quiet and rest and recovery. The stupid couch is waiting with open arms.

Love, hugs, and Expecting Miracles.

Holly

TO RED OR NOT TO RED
January 14, 2011

Now that chemo is over (well the infusions at least - still have some recovery to go), I wanted to have a little fun with this (not like I haven't been having fun up to this point). No money will be exchanged, but we can do an unofficial and fun only voting pool on the growth and color of my hair as it grows back.

Here's what the doctors are saying:

1. Color - could be red, could be darker (brown), a gray mix, or all gray.

2. Texture - could be curly, curlier (gads), or straight.

3. Growth - typically one to three months after chemo is when it begins to grow back, which would be sometime between mid-February and mid-April. Full growth will then happen over time. The average hair grows 1/2 inch a month. Do the math on your own.

Now those are their opinions... when you send in your votes, you can go from their suggestions or come up with your own ideas! No feelings will be hurt with what you pick - although for fun only - this is meant to be competitive!

1. What color will my hair be?
2. What texture will my hair be?
3. At a full growth out, what date will my hair be 1 inch long?

Send me your votes for those three questions... I'm hoping to get most of them in this long weekend while I'm recovering. But the official end date to cast your vote is midnight of 31 January. One vote per person.

The winners will be announced.... well... when it finally grows out!!!

Love, hugs, and getting my fabulous stylist Melissa queued up with some red dye just in case!

Holly

CHEMOGEDDON
January 17, 2011

I am a self-admitted rip-the-band-aid-off-fast kinda gal. Always have been. Always will be. I enjoy the anticipation up to the event, and the event itself (whatever said event may be)... but after the event, I'm on the road to the next one. Shut the door and move on. Lead, follow, or get out of my way. New Year's Day is traditionally the day when all of Christmas is boxed up and moved back to the attic. A once beautifully ornamented tree is now tagged, bagged, and tossed to the curb.

I survived my last infusion and the worst days that follow. I'm ready to move on. Chemo doesn't care. Chemo don't roll like that. The tree is out on the curb. But there are needles all over the living room carpet. And the vacuum cleaner doesn't work. Those pesky buggers have to be picked up one needle at a time. It's a bit of a mess, but I'll get every single one.

Love, hugs, and healing one day at a time.

Holly

CHAPTER 8 INVINCIBILITY
January 20, 2011

In the cancer handbook, they say this is the point of the journey where "invincibility" begins to rear its ugly head. At five foot nothing and the weight of a honey bee, I do better at playing the tough girl on daytime TV more so than reality will admit. Today presented a formidable opponent and a test to this new chapter.

Every old office building has its share of interesting inhabitants. This morning at 0700 one of them showed up at my doorstep at work and he had a bone to pick. A cockroach the size of a small farm animal. He caught me off guard, as I certainly wasn't expecting a visitor. The two other girls in my office were just as startled as I was. We huddled together, figuring there would be safety in a pack. We looked at each other. We looked at him. He looked back at us. "Step back ladies," I said, trying to protect my flock. I took off my boot. Not a snow boot. A black leather boot with three-inch heels. I lifted my arm brandishing the weapon to scare and intimidate.

Now... before I move forward, let me go back to another point in time when I encountered the same situation. At the moment my arm was raised with weapon in hand, I chickened out and instead turned and ran away screaming like a girl. Oh wait. I am one.

Today was different. Just as all of the brave warrior sisters before me who imparted their sage advice... "after you kick cancer's a** you will feel invincible," I did. There I was... weapon in hand. Ready to strike. He taunted me. He mocked me. He's been in this position before. He knows the deal. And he knows that he's going to win and live to see another day. But not this time. At that moment, the scars, the needles, the pain, and all of the rage against cancer (Tom

Morello is guest guitarist) came to the surface. Instead of being scared away, I was ready to rumble. And rumble I did. The girls were in shock that I actually went through with it, and cheered that I eliminated the foe. The office was safe again. Invincibility felt really good.

Love, hugs, and not jumping out of a plane any time soon.

Holly

VIVACIOUS

"Pick an adjective that describes yourself."

Vivacious was the first word that came to mind. Vivacious. Full of life. Ironic, considering I just finished chemotherapy, which killed everything inside me. With its death has come rebirth and regrowth. My bald head has no hair, but the brain inside tells humorous stories that make others laugh. I don't have eyebrows or eyelashes, but my eyes are wider, and more perceptive. I have scars on my chest, but my heart has never loved more. The top half of my fingernails are dead, but I can hold the hands of my fiancé and stepson. My feet still go numb sometimes, but I run five miles a week and am productive at work in my three-inch heels. I am vivacious. I am a cancer survivor. I am alive.

ILL TEMPERED TRIGONOMETRY
January 22, 2011

Monday begins the next phase of my cancer treatment. I transition my care from Virginia Hospital Center in Arlington to INOVA Alexandria Hospital since its closer to home to accommodate six weeks of daily radiation treatments. Now that scary evil chemo is over, I am excited as to what Monday will bring. They tell me to expect a 1.5 hour prep session that I have to lay still on a table and they have these "laser beams" (Mini Me, quit... nevermind) that will form some kind of trajectory so they can mark where to concentrate the radiation around the lymph nodes and the artist formerly known as the tumor. The doctor described it as one big trigonometry experiment. My initial thoughts wax curiosity over what kind of "laser beams" will they be? Will the doctor use sharks with fricken laser beams attached to their heads? Or maybe mutant sea bass?

My next thoughts go back to 11th grade Trigonometry, and despite getting an A in class, I wish I had paid more attention. All I remember is that it had to do something with a triangle and terms like sines, cosines, tangents, and hypotenuses.... and seriously... when the heck are you EVER going to use this information later in life? Gee... uh... only during important times like ensuring the high voltage radiation goes EXACTLY where it should and nowhere else. All I know is that in nine years I have ammunition when Stepson questions the relevance of higher math.

Love, hugs, and here's hoping my Doctor paid more attention in her Trig class... or at least doesn't use mutant crustacean to perform the procedure.

Holly

INOVA INK
January 24, 2011

I've always liked the idea of a tattoo, and always thought that they were super cool. But I could never bring myself to have something permanently inked on my body. Until now.

It was one of those nights. Carter and I started drinking at McConnells, and then stumbled over to Union Street. We were drinking whiskey and going shot for shot. I danced on the bar. Carter got into a fight. We found ourselves in front of the tattoo parlor. The next thing I know, Betty Boop and I are now forever one.

That is my "how I got my tattoo" story and I'm sticking to it.

Ok... ok... In reality, it went down like this... I'm half nakey laying on a table with my arm up in the air and a machine doing a 360 around me with the doctor and nurses running in and out of the room, and coming back and scribbling with sharpies all over my torso, which now closely resembles Rand McNally. The next thing I know, the doctor places a giant two-foot compass and protractor on my chest. I kid you not.

You could make a list of 5,839 items that would land on your boobies at some time throughout your life and I have to say...I never thought a compass and protractor would be one (two?) of them. After the trigonometry experiment was complete, Kat Von D came in and tattooed me up.

My rock star tattoo expectations fizzled. There was no dancing on the bar. Kat Von D is really Denise. My six rocking tats are barely noticeable. But I can add to the list of "things I've done in my lifetime"... having a protractor and compass on the girls. What a day.

Love, hugs, and check out the next episode of INOVA Ink on TLC.

Holly

LAUGH PRAY LOVE
January 27, 2011

Thank you to all of Team Bertone for your support and encouragement. I received quite a few emails over the last week that had similar commentary about laughing. And if you haven't commented directly to me about it, you may be thinking it... so here it is. Straight up.

According to my dear friend Marge, cancer cells die of embarrassment. Team Bertone's job is to pray and laugh and love, as that has been and will continue to help in my recovery. I hope you have enjoyed my emails and it's a huge blessing to have so many people cheering for me and it's been great therapy to write about this journey. So yes...please... laugh and enjoy. Then pay it forward in your own way.

Love, hugs, and keep smiling.

Holly

IT COMES IN OBAMA AND BRITNEY SPEARS TOO
February 1, 2011

The votes are in.

Color:
Red - 54%
Darker/Dark Red - 25%
Brown - 8%
Gray/White - 13%

Texture:
Straight - 27%
Wavey - 7%
Curly - 39%
Curlier - 7%

Date:
February - 3%
March - 18%
April - 37%
May - 19%
June - 18%
July - 5%

And great news... tiny intermittent stubble made an appearance on my head this week. When I showed Carter, we both started singing... Cha-Cha-Cha-Chia! So now it's a waiting game to see how it comes out. I will keep you posted with the "headline" news (tee hee) and who are the big winners.

Love, hugs, putting mud on my scalp and watching the sprouts grow.

Holly

CELEBRATING A SUPER CENTENNIAL SUNDAY
February 6, 2011

Two big events are happening today, and I was trying to figure out how to tie them together in today's musings. First on everyone's minds of course is the Super Bowl. Another big event today is the 100th birthday of President Ronald Reagan. What is the common bond you may ask? Passion.

The TV in our home is more of a Fox News and History Channel TV and I don't think it even knows what ESPN is. But we will still be watching the Super Bowl (er commercials... get the Doritos... get the Doritos...). I don't really care who wins (I hope your team does - go team!). But I will be cheering for the Green Bay Packer... fans. These are people who love their team so much, they wear giant cheese wedges on their heads. They are so crazy about their team that in a hospital in Wisconsin, they are putting itty bitty cheese heads on their newborn babies. SERIOUSLY? As insane as they are, I appreciate their passion, and their penchant for headwear.

Which brings me to the other celebration today. As a child coming of age in the '80's, President Reagan was "My President." While I didn't really understand politics at the time, watching and listening to President Reagan on TV was like hearing a story from my grandfather. I learned about Reaganomics in school. I remember "tear down this wall," and in 2005 spent a day in Germany traveling to Berlin just to see the remainder of the wall. But the President Reagan quote for today (actually taken from a poem from John Magee) is about passion, something this man exhibited his entire life. When Space Shuttle Challenger blew up (25 years ago last week), he commented, "The future doesn't belong to the fainthearted, it belongs to the brave..."

What are you passionate about? Are you chasing it? Or do you need to find it? What walls are you tearing down to create your future?

Love, hugs, wearing fabulous headwear, and looking through to the other side.

Go team! And get those Doritos!!!!!

Holly

MONDAY VERSION 3.0
February 7, 2011

With the first week of radiation under my belt and 30 treatments to go, it doesn't hurt, it's certainly not as bad as chemo, it doesn't make me sick, but I am now narcoleptic. They said the fatigue should kick in around the third week or so. Wow, if this isn't fatigue, I don't want to meet its big brother. Just another something I have to deal with, but the biggest thing for me right now... I want my body back and I've been pushing myself hard in the gym to find it again.

3.0 miles. As seen this morning on the treadmill for the first time in... wow... I can't even remember. Oh wait, I can. The last time I ran three miles was at the first chemo treatment when I was all doped up on steroids. Ok, Ok... outside of being under the influence of a performance enhancing substance legally prescribed by a physician, I can't remember the last time I made it three miles. I still can't run the whole way but it's a big milestone. Tomorrow I'll try to actually stay awake during my run.

Love, hugs, and enjoying nap time.

Holly

THE GREATEST OF THESE IS YOU
February 14, 2011

Love is patient. Love is kind.

Love is an army of family, friends, and complete strangers who have taken time out of their day to pray, send cards, emails, texts, homemade cards, YouTube videos, and care packages. Love dropped off food, helped around the house, and keeps me updated on all things not cancer related. Love is two little girls I never met who gave up their portable DVD player for long chemo days. Love shaves the hair off a future daughter-in-law's head.

Love is being taught fortitude my entire life to conquer challenges such as these. And a story of a man in a row boat who goes and gets.

Love always protects, always trusts, always hopes, always perseveres.

Love is on one knee proposing 48 hours after my breast cancer diagnosis. Love grows stronger every day despite two big scars and a bald coconut head.

Love is innocent. Love knows that watching Sponge Bob cartoons together on the couch will solve all of the problems in the world.

Love never fails.
Holly

SOMETIMES YOU FEEL LIKE A NUT
February 17, 2011

...sometimes you don't. One of the most frustrating aspects about this cancer thing is the lack of choice and control. You will have this appointment at this time. You will be on this drug. You will have this treatment. This week introduced another specialist and an even bigger list of Do's and Don'ts as I venture into living a new life after breast cancer treatment with lymphodema prevention. No restrictions that are too earth shattering or life altering, but the fact remains, this ain't no over-and-done thing. I'm in it for life. It is a good thing the medical professionals guide you along their expert chosen path. But it breeds a sense of helplessness. And especially at a time when I was feeling good and seeing progress for the first time in M-O-N-T-H-S... yesterday's appointment took a little wind out of my sail.

My new hospital, whether they know it or not, remedies a piece of this in their own little way. And every day I'm there, I look forward to making a choice. The choice is all mine. No doctor is leading or guiding this decision. I have a choice of where to park my car. Some days when it's cold or rainy, I drive to the door and let the free valet park my car. Some days, I pull into one of the closer "Reserved for Cancer Patient" spots and feel like royalty. The last few days it's been so nice outside, I parked across the street in the back of the lot to enjoy the extra walk in the warm sun.

I know it doesn't sound like much. But where I park my car is one of the few pieces of this cancer thing that I can control. And today when I came home, instead of taking a nap I took a short run in the beautiful sun and 65 degree weather. And all is well in the world.

Love, hugs, and I hate coconut.

Holly

PAIN IS WEAKNESS LEAVING THE BODY
February 19, 2011

Today marks the 66th anniversary of the beginning of the month long Battle of Iwo Jima, the battle that resulted in one of the most famous and recognizable photographs in history, and a battle that became USMC and WWII legend. For those of you who don't know my background, I spent quite a few years working in Quantico. I spent mornings before work running on the trails and obstacle courses. After work, I taught spin class in the USMC gym... I instructed military and civilian classes, and Unit PT. I also was extremely honored to be the token civilian on the USMC Quantico mountain bike team in 2005 and 2006. And trust me, while training with the Marines, I was in the best shape of my life, and had my best ever mountain bike season, even after breaking a rib in the peak of spring training.

A while back, a friend of Carter's gave us matching USMC t-shirts with a slogan, "Pain is Weakness Leaving the Body." For whatever reason, that t-shirt was on my back all week at the gym (stinky!). This week has also been the beginning of a turning point that despite being in a constant state of exhaustion, I can actually feel myself starting to heal, and feel my body starting to change back to the way it should feel. The last two days after radiation treatment, I bypassed the couch for my daily nap and laced up the Nikes for a couple jogs in the sun and 65-70 degree weather (ok.. ok...I confess... I did still take a nap afterwards). This week, it's moving forward one step at a time. And letting the weakness leave my body.

Love, hugs, and Godspeed to all of our troops.

Holly

IT'S 5 O'CLOCK SOMEWHERE IN THE WORLD
February 21, 2011

Location - on my head. As spotted this morning - a 5 o'clock shadow. Carter has already dubbed me baby duckling, and I'm sure more fun nicknames will be forthcoming. It doesn't have color yet...

Ron White (one of the blue collar comedy guys) said, "I believe that when life gives you lemons, you should make lemonade... and try to find someone whose life has given them vodka, and have a party." I'm not sure if I'm the lemon or the vodka, but it's 5 o'clock somewhere and there's a party happening on my head.

Cheers. Salute. Salud. Egeszsegedre.

Holly

YARD SALE
February 23, 2011

yard sale *n.* (from skiing, snowboarding, mountain biking) a horrendous crash that leaves all your various "wares" -- water bottles, pump, tool bag, gloves, poles, etc. -- scattered as if on display for sale.

This cancer thing left me with some interesting side effects to deal with. While none of this is anywhere as bad as chemo, the annoying factor is almost comical.

Chest... Right on schedule, my fair red head skin is showing signs of its daily radiation bombardment. Supposedly, some women have nice glowing tans from radiation on that area. I, of course, was hoping for that option, especially considering I'm heading to the waterpark in another month. Nope - no such luck. I get the itchy, scratchy, blotchy, irritated, rashy kind. Oh joy. In addition to my lucky fin, two scars, and six tattoos, that entire quadrant is now covered in a rash that the prescribed lotions and potions won't ease (and all very "normal" according to the doctor). I don't know how to describe it other than I am coming out of my skin and I have four more weeks of this fun. Cue the old camp song... "itchy itchy scratchy scratchy oooey oooey owey owey wish it go away."

Face... still dealing with the remnants of the taxotere, I woke up this morning not just to watery eyes, but to puffy, swollen eyes. No makeup for me today. Oh wait... I can still paint on my eyebrows. The plucking incident of 1999 left me with sparse eyebrows to begin with so I'm used to filling them in. But with chemo, I lost a lot of what little was left so now it's an all on assault of paint while channeling Lucille Ball.

Head... Carter and I inspect my head every day for new hair growth.

While I'm sick of covering up my head and am ready to go free-balding in public, there is also the balance of dignity, vanity, bravery, and social appropriateness. Carter's latest description was akin to me spreading glue on my head and then covering it with dryer lint. And we're not talking about the second load of towels - this is more like the dryer lint from the polyester load. Hence today's nickname, "DL." Better than "dog with mange" - which is what my head looked like when I lost my hair.

I think God gives you exhaustion at this point so you are just too tired to care how you look - rashy chest, swollen puffy eyes, and dryer lint for hair. It was one of those days where I was so tired I couldn't get out of bed and looked an absolute hot mess. But... I made it to work, I had a great run, a little kinder bueno for a snack, and I got to pick Stepson up at school. And aside from not having naptime today, all is well in the world.

Love, hugs, picking up a few more pieces, and going to bed early tonight.

Holly

THE PLAGUE
February 25, 2011

It is a rite of passage every winter for most folks. At some point when the temperatures drop, the germs take over. And you get the plague... whether it's a cold or flu or stomach or sinus or general malaise... we all go through it. We can't predict when it will happen to us, but it's an almost certainty that it will.

From the time this cancer thing started, I haven't been real-sick, only dealing with treatment side effects of cancer-sick. Which I find completely ironic... I'm dealing with being the sickest as I have ever been in my life, but I've managed to stay healthy throughout this entire time. In the last seven months, I haven't taken one real bonafide "sick day" at work. In the last seven months while my body has been broken and violated and my immune system completely compromised, I've been blessed to stay healthy. But it was only a matter of time.

Earlier this week, I thought it was normal fatigue and side effects from radiation. I wasn't even thinking about being sick. As in for real sick. So I kept going... and going... and then not so much. My run of good health had officially ended. I joined the masses in participating in the winter ritual of having the plague. And after months of closely monitoring and calculating the unknown and unexpected side effects from treatment, it was comforting to go back to the basics - Netti Rinse, NyQuil, mindless TV, and lots of sleep.

Fortunately I'm feeling better today than yesterday, but I'm following doctors orders and doing nothing but resting.

Love, hugs, and back to the stupid couch.
Holly

BEAUTY IS WHERE YOU FIND IT
February 26, 2011

First of all... yes, I have been resting. Despite popular opinion, I do know how to hit the stop button every once in a while. :)

I always try to leave the house put together in respectable clothing and makeup. With being sick the last few days, I did not put on any makeup. And then I caught a glimpse of myself in the mirror. And noticed that I'm missing something on the right side of my face. Now, I fully realize that I lost a lot and I've had to fill in to the point of painting on new eyebrows, but it was mostly on autopilot and I didn't realize the severity of it until now. I have 12 lonely eyebrow hairs. T-W-E-L-V-E. In the cancer world, this is when you go from looking human to looking alien. One of the biggest compliments I received recently was, "at least you didn't lose your eyebrows." Oh God bless that gave me the biggest smile. Thanks goodness for great makeup and great makeup skills! The American Cancer Society puts on a class I attended a few months ago when this all started called "Look Good Feel Good" and they show you how to apply makeup during treatment (and you get to keep about $200 in designer makeup... woo hoo Chanel is the ultimate breast cancer booby prize!!!). Between that and my dear Michelle helping me through the plucking incident of 1999, I have the tools I need to successfully recreate great brows. Fortunately, my eyelashes didn't sustain too much damage and I'll be wearing mascara again real soon.

Breast cancer has taken away enough aspects of my femininity. I'm not going to let this one bother me, especially since it's an easy fix (and who knows... maybe they will grow back???). I will never again see the Brooke Shields eyebrows of my youth. But I'm now in great company. Think of all of the beautiful icons of the past who had thin, defined brows: Greta Garbo, Lucille Ball, Rita Hayworth, Jean

Harlow, Ginger Rogers, Mae West, Judy Garland. Ladies with an attitude...strike a pose there's nothing to it.

Love, hugs, and in my sick throaty voice... come up and see me sometime.

Holly

NIP TUCK DROPS AND ROLL
March 1, 2011

If you told me at the beginning of this cancer thing that I would be seeing a plastic surgeon, it would have sounded very plausible. Brave warrior sisters of the past stood up and fought Congress and now if you lose a breast or two to breast cancer surgery, it is law that insurance will cover the reconstruction. Go girls! Although today... different part of the anatomy. Today, I saw an eye plastic surgeon. I didn't even realize they exist. The tearing I've been experiencing from the taxotere is a pretty serious side effect and needs to be taken care of without delay.

After a quick consult with his assistant, I sit in the exam chair and watch the commercials on the little TV of all the different procedures this type of plastic surgeon can do (in the plastic surgery business they call this an "upsale"). Botox will NOT be a part of my 40,000 mile tune up. I'm not sure what type of bona fides to look for in an eye plastic surgeon. This isn't LA, but they say Washington, DC is like the Hollywood for ugly people. So I'm guessing that being named as one of The Washingtonian's best plastic surgeons, that's good enough street cred for me.

WARNING... if you are faint of heart or on certain types of medications... skip to the next paragraph!!!!! The procedure began with a few innocent drops. And then Dr. Evil put eight needles in the tear ducts of my eyes. Yes. EIGHT. Four in each eye. Words. Cannot. Describe. Oh. My. God. After bamboo torture came the water boarding. The procedure was completed by the tear ducts being flushed with a saline rinse. As I'm laying mostly inverted and he's pouring the saline rinse into my eyes, it transports down into my throat and chokes me. Someone please call the Secretary of Defense as there are some torture laws that need to be updated. I also have a prescription for drops I need to use for the next two weeks, and I have a follow up appointment in a month. I'm not sure if this procedure was supposed to be "THE" procedure to take care of the problem, or if this was just an evaluation to determine if I need another procedure. I was too scared to ask and ignorance is bliss. But when I go back, I will be in full body armor.

The super cool thing about it... and especially for those of you who are addicted to the Netti Rinse will appreciate this...the results are like 100 times better... my sinuses have never been more clear.

Love, hugs, and breathing easy.

Holly

LET IT GROW
March 2, 2011

"Freedom has a scent, like the top of a new born baby's head." (U2 - Miracle Drug)

My head is not that of a new born baby. But it is newborn. Every day it grows, and the progress albeit small, is visible. It is still too early to distinguish a specific color.

I hit my cracking point this week with covering my head, and I started to free-bald it. Probably a week or two too early. But I don't care anymore. I will still cover my head for certain occasions, but for everyday living, it's now out there.

Love, hugs, and enjoying freedom.

Holly

60 DAYS
March 3, 2011

Anyone who has crossed my path lately has heard me say, "I have too much going on. I don't have time for cancer." Today... I sprint out of the office, drive to the jewelry store to pick up my wedding band, drive to the hospital for treatment (and oh btw I had to stay extra long as the Dr. had to prep the area for the next phase of radiation - The Boost), drive to the medical store and get fitted for my lymphedema prevention sleeve (need to wear it only when flying on an airplane and exercising - fortunately not all day long), drive home, pick up Carter, and then drive to the courthouse (no nap for me!!!!). Oh and then come back home and bake a cake for Stepson's birthday. Thank goodness for leftovers tonight!

Carter and I picked up the marriage license today. The marriage license expires in 60 days, so we're in the window to tie the knot on 31 March.

When Carter proposed, I was excited and scared. I was excited for our future lives together, but scared about this cancer thing. Scared about my health. Scared about what cancer would do to our relationship. Scared about the unknown. Since then, our lives have been turned upside down and both of us have been tested every day.

When Carter proposed, I looked like any normal happy bride-to-be should look. Neither of us expected me to be bald on our wedding day. We've watched each other deal with this cancer thing, and we've learned a lot about each other. We've been through more together in the last eight months then some couples deal with in a lifetime. When we walked into the courthouse today, it was with the same emotion as one would have picking up the dry cleaning. No panic. No cold feet. We're both at the point where this is such a sure thing

71

it's like it already happened.

After the wedding, another 60 day countdown begins. In June, Carter will deploy overseas for four months, so once we get back from the familymoon, the clock is ticking to get all of our married affairs in order before he leaves. Thank goodness at that point, I won't have this cancer thing getting in the way.

Love, hugs, crossing things off my list, and taking it a day at a time.

Holly

THEY SAY IT'S YOUR BIRTHDAY
March 5, 2011

At the same time as I'm battling cancer, I'm also preparing to be a new wife and stepmother. Getting married (again) is a big step, and inheriting a stepson and being responsible for the upbringing of a young child who is not genetically mine is even more daunting. Watching Stepson grow and mature over the last couple years has been a very rewarding experience, and I'm learning my new place in the world of being a stepmom.

"Prepare the child for the path, not the path for the child." We live in a current society of raising our children that everyone is a winner and life is always perfect, and protecting our children from the bad things in life. Whatever happened to the good ole days of sucking on lead paint in the crib and 10 kids being thrown in the back of the station wagon without restraint and running around outside all day without parental supervision?

The reality is that life happens whether you want it to or not. And life isn't always rainbows and butterflies. I want to walk in a path of strength and grace and be a good example. I want to teach Stepson to be courageous and compassionate, have good manners, and arm him with the tools to be a survivor when life doesn't go as planned. I also want to teach him to appreciate the Beatles, despite the fact that his father favors the Stones.

Happy #8 to my #1 buddy. May the next 88 years be full of goodness and happiness and I promise you my best.

Love, hugs, and eating cake.

Holly

KUBLER, ROSS, AND BERTONE
March 7, 2011

I want to make sure my parents get their money's worth from my BA in Psychology... so I'm updating the Kubler Ross model of grief. You know how when something bad happens (death, illness, etc), you go through the stages of grief... Denial (nothing is wrong), Anger (mad at the world), Bargaining (I'll do anything), Depression (being sad), and Acceptance (all is well). Well...I think the model for cancer is a little different. Having breast cancer is like going through the Cycle of the 7 Dwarfs.

Doc - You pretty much see one every day.

Bashful - The first few weeks at diagnosis I was completely bashful to show the girls and then transitioned to wishing I had a dollar for every time I had to undress...

Sneezy - The first sustaining side effect I had with taxotere was a runny nose and watery eyes.

Dopey - Chemo brain. Need I say more?

Sleepy - Pretty much my world every day for the last few months, and now it's worse with radiation. This sh*t makes you T-I-R-E-D!!!!!

Grumpy - What I am when I don't get enough sleep. See above. Pray for Carter.

Happy - The ideal state. Where I want to be and strive to be.

Love, hugs, and whistling while I work. Holly

BROKEN

We were positive through cancer. We laughed through cancer. But I still had my share of tears and a few meltdowns of epic proportion. These very private conversations became defining moments of our relationship, and also breaking through dealing with cancer. I'm sharing them with you because I want you to know you are not alone. It's natural to feel this way. It's ok to feel this way. But you have to fight through it and get over it.

I don't even remember what set me off this time.

"I don't know why you want to be with me. I'm bald and I'm missing part of my breast and I have big scars and it's not fair to you. You deserve to be with a beautiful fiancé and wife. You deserve to be with a woman who is..."

Carter wouldn't let me finish the sentence. "Don't even say I deserve to be with a woman who is whole. You are whole, and I love you just the way you are. If I come back from Afghanistan missing an arm or a leg, would you love me any less?"

"I would probably love you even more."

No more conversation was needed. The tears eventually stopped.

RAINY DAYS AND THURSDAYS
ALWAYS GET ME DOWN
March 10, 2011

Yesterday was Ash Wednesday, the beginning of Lent. I've never been a big giver-upper-for-Lent kinda person. I started off my day joking around that I was giving up cancer for Lent, which I think is perfectly legit. And far better to give up cancer than Girl Scout cookies I mean come on who are we kidding here, right?

I don't think it's an accident... but my time for radiation is right after the newbie slot. The newbie slot is a set time every day reserved for new patients for their final measurement before they begin their radiation treatment. So when the women come back into the changing room to wait for their meeting with the doctor, I'm sitting there, ready to go in for my treatment. And we chat for a few minutes. Every day. It's a different woman every day. But really... it's the same woman and the same conversation. Wide eyed and a bit scared of the unknown. "Whatcha in for?" I always ask to break the ice. And I always give her the "everything will be ok" smile.

I'm now the vet. I'm now the "been there, done that." And without even realizing it, every day of my radiation treatment, I've been paying it forward for the next woman. It's been one of those weeks for me. Part Murphy's Law where everything hits at once, part cancer, part being generally miserable. And when Mamma's miserable, everyone is miserable (pray for Carter). I'm at the point now where I'm over this cancer thing and despite being one of those weeks, I don't need to share my grumptastic self with everyone else.

Yes. Cancer has worn me down. I'm exhausted. I'm beat up. I'm miserable. Did I mention I'm exhausted? I have seven treatments to go and I'm on the home stretch, and I have a wedding and familymoon to plan for and look forward to. I can't and I won't let cancer or anything else get in the way of my happiness. So I'm giving up being grumpy for Lent. For real.

Love, hugs, and the sun will come out tomorrow.

Holly

NEW OLD NEW NORMAL
March 11, 2011

The time leading up to the initial diagnosis, and especially the first month or so after diagnosis was life changing and devastating news to deal with. After processing way too much information and dealing with way more than I had to, I started hearing about "new normal."

New normal is the term that doctors and patients use to describe settling into the cancer routine and living a "normal" life with cancer. It's more than acceptance; it's a new routine, and a new way of life. It's making all of the bad parts of cancer a normal way of life. New normal is a double-edged sword.

There is the place where I hated new normal and all I wanted is for life to go back to the way it was. But new normal is a place you need to get to pretty quickly. New normal is necessary. New normal is survival. Once settled into new normal, everything feels better, and a level of sanity and routine come back. I let new normal enter our lives as quickly as I could, because it was much easier to cope in new normal. It felt good.

Chemo is over, and I'm almost through radiation. It's time. I want to get out of new normal as quickly as possible. The last month, there were several events that helped to take us out of new normal and back to old normal. I wore my wig, and Carter and I went out to dinner without cancer being a topic of conversation. We picked out our wedding rings. I spent an afternoon with some girlfriends. I ran outside. We re-instituted Monday box taco night.

I want our lives and routines to go back to old normal, but I hope that cancer changed a part of me, and I want to figure out how I'm going to use this gift. Plus, there is the lifetime aspect of checkups and lifestyle modifications. So going back to old normal is more of an ambition to find a new old new normal. Or some nice balance in between.

Love, hugs, and finding my way.

Holly

38TH PARALLEL
March 12, 2011

Between chemo and radiation, my body has formed its own lines of demarcation. Chemo gave my fingernails this disgusting orange-brown color, and once the doctors didn't want to check my fingernails for damage any more, I started painting them to hide how gross they looked. Well, after taking off the nail polish this week, I noticed a line exactly half way through each fingernail. North of the parallel, my nails are still under communist rule. South of the parallel, they are free and happy and have a normal healthy pink color.

Onto "the quadrant." Radiation treatment is given not just to my lucky fin, but to the entire front, side, and back, ergo... the quadrant. As I said before, radiation did not give me a healthy glow, but more of the itchy rashy side effect. Well, thank goodness for precision. There is literally a visible border that defines the entire irritated treatment area, like a reverse bathing suit mark on a bad sun burn. And the line follows the permanent tattoos and the daily sharpie marks. It is absolutely comical, when you think this all came to fruition because of a giant protractor and compass on my boobies.

I'm finally making the transition from my body being a hot mess, to visible signs of where the hot mess ends and the new Holly begins.

Love, hugs, and drawing lines for world domination.

Holly

IT PLACES THE LOTION IN THE BASKET
March 14, 2011

I must say that between two hospitals, three doctors, two patient navigators, a gazillion nurses, and the American Cancer Society... I'm not without an abundance of pamphlets and brochures briefing me on all aspects of cancer and cancer treatment. As I near the end of my treatment journey, I'm reading about post-treatment depression. These pamphlets are warning me that after my body has been broken and violated for months on end and giving up all of my vacation and leave time at work to either be in the hospital, at an appointment, or home sick, that I will now be sad and miss going through treatments and all of the attention at the hospital. SERIOUSLY?

That after...
1 biopsy
1 surgery
2 mammograms
2 scars
6 tests
6 tattoos
16 hours of draino
25 needles
34 radiation treatments
+ 5 years of yet another drug

... that somehow I'm going to miss all of this? Again... SERIOUSLY? (and keep in mind that I fell on the easy side of the cancer street, so these numbers are very low compared to most cancer treatments).

Are you telling me that in addition to having to deal with: abdominal pain, bone pain, breathing problems, bruises, chemo brain, constipation, cough, cramping, diarrhea, dry mouth, dry skin, fatigue,

GI issues, hair loss, hot flashes, insomnia, joint pain, menopause, metallic taste, mouth sores, muscle pain, nausea, neuropathy, nosebleeds, numbness, rashes, runny nose, shortness of breath, sunburn, taste changes, walking farts, watery eyes, and weakness...... that we need to add Stockholm Syndrome to the list of side effects? Someone please call the American Cancer Society so that they can update their brochures.

My medical team is amazing, and they have given me the best treatments in the world. But let me make this crystal clear. I'm not going to miss all of the treatments and appointments. I have more important things to occupy my time. I'm looking forward to our wedding and familymoon. All I want is to get out of the well and for my life to go back to normal.

Love, hugs, and... where's Precious?

Holly

BEWARE THE IDES OF MARCH
March 15, 2011

Appropriately on the Ides of March, my body has betrayed me once again. The level of fatigue and exhaustion has gone from manageable to... indescribable.

I keep thinking of one of my favorite lines from one of my favorite movies... Finding Nemo.

"Dory: Hey there, Mr. Grumpy Gills. When life gets you down do you wanna know what you've gotta do?

Marlin: No I don't wanna know.

Dory: Just keep swimming. Just keep swimming. Just keep swimming, swimming, swimming."

This is a level of existence that I never knew possible. I just hope I can keep it up for one more week.

Love, hugs, and et tu Brute?

Holly

COLLATERAL DAMAGE
March 16, 2011

Today I felt slightly better; however I knew I was on borrowed time. I had two appointments at the hospital, and despite leaving work a little early, my hope was for the planets to align that I could get home in time for a nap before I left to pick up Stepson at school.

Both my appointment and radiation went as planned, and slightly early, and I was ecstatic and on a mission - homeward bound for a much needed nap.

I pulled a Clark Kent and changed in record time and it was one swift motion to leave the dressing room and head down the hallway and out of the hospital. Clack-clack-clack-clack-clack the three-inch heels were pulling double time on the linoleum floor. I turned the corner... and ran head on and smack into... one of the lab techs. He was a decent sized guy. And as he stumbled, he all but took out the tiny elderly lady he was escorting.

I was insanely embarrassed and horrified that in my haste, this dear lady was close to being a casualty. I apologized profusely. He said something about watching it and she was a bit in shock. I made sure they were both ok (and they were - no harm, no foul) and said something to the effect of I have exactly 90 minutes to get home, take a quick nap, and pick up my stepson.

I don't have time for cancer. Please forgive me. I think they did. I hope they did. It's a sad state of affairs when my haste for naptime causes me to run down kind people in the hallway.

Yes, I got my nap. And yes, I picked Stepson up on time. And yes, I'm glad the boys are now at a Cub Scout meeting because I am drinking a glass of wine and I am one with the stupid couch and nearing bed time and it's only 7:15. Shhhhhh.....

Love, hugs, and countdown to more ZZZZZs.

Holly

KISS ME I'M IRISH
March 17, 2011

May the road rise up to meet you.
May the wind always be at your back.
May the sun shine warm upon your face,
And rains fall soft upon your fields.
And until we meet again,
May God hold you in the palm of His hand.

Love, hugs, and drinking Guinness.

Holly

PS - Yep... I wore the green wig to work.

INSTANT KARMA'S GONNA GET YOU
March 18, 2011

Today was another workhospitalnappickupStepsonmakedinner days, so even though it was a nice day outside, I pulled into the front parking lot of the hospital, hoping to get a close spot. Ok follow me here. There is a car in the driving lane parked perpendicular to the parked cars with the driver STANDING OUTSIDE THE CAR (important to note). The minivan in front of me stops beside the car for no reason at all, so I'm blocked in. After a few seconds I give a honk and the security guard comes up to the minivan and tells them to move along. They do. I pull into the empty spot in front of the parked car (still parked in the driving lane and the driver is still STANDING OUTSIDE OF HIS CAR).

I get out of my car. Dude comes running over at me screaming that I took his parking space that he was going to back into it (like maybe tomorrow?????). I didn't even have time to react... the security guard runs over to the dude and steps in and starts yelling at him..."She's a cancer patient. She can park here. Look... she doesn't have any hair. She has her cancer center ID badge. She gets this spot. She has priority. You go park somewhere else." (I ran two miles this morning... but hey if you want to come to my defense and play the cancer card on my behalf... go for it my man).

I said a very quick and quiet thank you to the security guard and exit stage right to the hospital. I certainly wasn't about to get in the middle of that one. I'm beginning to think that being a cancer patient is hazardous to your health.

Love, hugs, and we all shine on... like the moon and the stars and the sun.
Holly

WHISPER TO A SCREAM
March 20, 2011

For some bizarre reason, the word "cancer" cannot be spoken in a normal voice. People always start with a pause, and then the look, and then it's whispered. It's almost if you say the word "cancer" out loud that you will catch it. Or it's a big secret. Ummm... I kinda already know that I have cancer and it's not contagious. Hushed tones are not necessary.

There are differences in opinion when one becomes a cancer survivor. Most people agree you become a survivor at diagnosis. But after living through eight months of h-e-double-hockey-sticks, the word survivor takes on a whole new meaning as you come to the end of treatment. And as quiet as cancer is spoken, survivorship is shouted from the roof tops.

With one treatment to go, I attended a Survivor's Conference this weekend. Eight magic words in August and eight months later, I have two new families. One I'm marrying into. One I fought hard every day to be a part of. For the rest of my life, I will be a cancer survivor. And I have an amazing new family of other cancer survivors. It's an instant bond. It's understanding and encouragement for the newly diagnosed. It's a celebration of life with fellow survivors.

I go about my day and do my thing. But in the process, I've been pulled aside several times at work by folks who just learned of a loved one who was diagnosed with breast cancer. And most of them I barely know, and I am honored that they feel comfortable with me to share their worry and concern, and ask very personal questions. What does this (fill in the blank) mean? How should I act? What can I do to help? How did you find out? What did you go through?

What is worse - chemo or radiation?

Survivorship is an honor. Survivorship is a privilege. JFK summed up Luke 12:48 quite well, "With privilege comes responsibility." Survivorship is my gift and my responsibility.

Love, hugs, and forever your warrior sister.

Holly

IT'S NOT YOU. IT'S ME.
March 21, 2011

Dear Cancer -

We've had our share of good times and bad. You made me bruised. You gave me scars. We shared needles. You gave me a rash. You made me bald. I now have six tattoos on my body to remind me of that crazy time we had together. Because of you, I will be on a special drug therapy for the next five years. It's time we went our separate ways. It's not you. It's me. Oh wait. It IS you.

"SO WHAT
I'M STILL A ROCK STAR
I GOT MY ROCK MOVES
AND I DON'T NEED YOU
AND GUESS WHAT
I'M HAVING MORE FUN
AND NOW THAT WE'RE DONE
I'M GOING TO SHOW YOU
TONIGHT
I'M ALRIGHT
I'M JUST FINE
AND YOU'RE A TOOL
SO
SO WHAT
I'M STILL A ROCK STAR
I GOT MY ROCK MOVES
AND I DON'T WANT YOU TONIGHT"
(Thanks Pink!)

I wish this breakup would have fit on a post-it note.

NEXT STEPS
March 22, 2011

Over my career, I've had to make a lot of PowerPoint briefings, and my favorite slide is always the last one, regardless of the content of the brief, it's titled, "next steps." Now that treatment is over, I've had a lot of questions about my recovery and the way ahead.

First of all... no celebration yesterday for my last day of treatment. I went home and took a long nap and spent the remainder of the night on the couch. Party on. Excellent.

The extreme fatigue should subside in about 2 weeks, and I should "feel better" in a month. I told my doctor yesterday we need to be more aggressive with that timeline... I need to feel better in time for the wedding/familymoon next week. The loosey goosey standard seems to be that "recovery" takes as long as your entire treatment. So going through eight months of treatment, my body "should" recover in about eight months. But it's not like one day it's over and you are fine. Recovery is now a part of life.

There will be frequent check-ups in the first year. I have three doctors I will be seeing every six months until they tell me I can see them once a year. Then it's once a year for life. Same with the mammogram - every six months for five years. I'm on tamoxifen for five years, with two months already under my belt.

There may be random latent side effects that may or may not occur. This much treatment and this many chemicals are not without precautions for long term side effects, including additional cancers. It's the price that must be paid and the cost of doing business, and worth the risk.

And there will always be the question mark following me around. I will try my best to ignore it.

I want life to be as normal as possible, but there will be some changes. There are some minor adjustments I have made due to the issues in my arm...I carry my bag on my left shoulder and I need to be cautious about how much I lift and I have to wear the sleeve when I exercise and fly in a plane and be extra careful of infections and bug bites. Before cancer, I ate pretty healthy and exercised, but it will be amped up from now on. And finally, I want to pay it forward. I'm not sure what that means at this point, but I know the right doors will open. That's the exciting part. The new journey of life after cancer.

Love, hugs, and taking my next steps one at a time.

Holly

SOMETHING OLD, SOMETHING NEW
March 27, 2011

Back in August, when Carter proposed, I never expected my wedding day would be like this. Every bride wants to be beautiful on her wedding day. Every bride wants her wedding day to be perfect. The eight months leading up to their wedding day, most brides are making fun plans and trying on dresses and picking out flowers and invitations. The eight months leading up to my wedding day, I had chemo and radiation. The eight months leading up to their wedding day, most brides and grooms pick out an exotic location for a honeymoon. We picked a good hospital and the best surgery option. Carter and I certainly got a head start on the "for worse" and "in sickness." If we can survive cancer together, we can make it through anything. Going forward, we pray there is much more "for better" and "in health" in store for us.

Breast cancer is a triple threat as it typically takes away the three things that outwardly define a woman - her hair, her breasts, her fertility.

There have been moments throughout this journey that were tough blows to the self-esteem. This weekend I did a final prep and tried on my wedding dress and bathing suit. The mirror was cruel. For a moment, I was something blue. I'm getting married without hair, eyebrows, or eyelashes. I'm getting married with 2 scars and a lucky fin. On my wedding day, I will have fingernails that are discolored and dead and missing the top 1/4 that I'm not sure a manicure can fix. I am the exact same weight today as I was before this cancer thing, but during chemo I netted a cumulative gain/loss of 50 pounds in four months. Despite being faithful to the gym throughout treatment, the fluctuations took a toll on my body.

I took a deep breath and borrowed some strength.

I had to let go of the something old and embrace the something new. Beauty is not my bald head, but it is my brains which are smart and have the ability to make others laugh. Beauty is not my scars and lucky fin, but my heart underneath and the ability to love. And beauty is not chemical menopause, but committing to raising my new stepson and taking care of my new family.

I spent the last eight months kicking cancer's a**. I am a survivor. And my wedding day will be perfect, because my boys will be by my side, and because they never left.

Love, hugs, and ready to say I do.

Holly

THE RETURN OF DOCTOR EVIL
April 10, 2011

After the torture session at my last appointment with Dr. Evil, I wasn't sure what to expect at the follow up. I was too scared to ask if the eight twisting needles in my tear ducts followed by the saline rinse water boarding was "the procedure" or just a test to determine if I was a candidate for "the procedure." Ignorance was pure bliss.

Right before the wedding, I went back to Dr. Evil to discuss my response to the torture, and then options. None of which are good.

Door #1 - Do nothing. My personal favorite. If the condition does not worsen, I'm fine and all is well in the world. But... if the condition does worsen.... I'm looking at...

Door #2 - A glass tube implant in my tear duct area that is a super invasive surgery requiring drilling out a small piece of bone (like drilling any piece of bone is good????) for a permanent solution but with a slippery tube that has the chance of moving or coming out and having to go back every few months for placement. Oh and if I sneeze too hard, the glass tube might be shot through my nose and across the room. Think about that happening in a meeting at work.

Door #3 - A minimally invasive surgery (note - it's called SURGERY... not a procedure) I will sleep through in which Dr. Evil implants a long wire into and through my tear ducts and down my nose. I have to leave it in place for three months and I will have trouble breathing and I quote "it's pretty miserable to have it in but worth it when it comes out." I dared to ask how it comes out.... "oh that's the easy part I just pull it down through your nose." Cringeworthy.

I love a doctor who tries to have a sense of humor. When I asked Dr. Evil if I should chance not doing anything, he said his crystal ball doesn't have the most recent software upgrade. Sigh... but he did say all of his cancer patients who had this same surgery had remarkable improvement and no complications. And he is a Washingtonian Best Doctor. I still have plenty of time to make up my mind.

Love, hugs and trading my tear ducts for the Deal of the Day.

Holly

AND THE WINNER IS...
May 31, 2011

This weekend finally hit a major milestone.

One inch.
Dark red.
Curly.

Since we are dealing with hair and a margin of error... there are several winners.

It's funny... at a mere inch long...my hair is already showing signs of being strong willed and rebellious. I can only hope as my strength returns to its pre-cancerous self, that I follow my hair's lead.

Love, hugs, and thanks for playing!

Holly

OVER THE HILL
July 9, 2011

"You don't have a choice in how you are going to die, but you do have a choice in how you are going to live." I know this is a famous quote, but no clue who said it.

Recovery is almost more difficult than treatment. During treatment, I had an opponent. I had a very tangible foe to battle every day. Now during recovery, I'm still just as tired and worn down. But I'm not fighting cancer any more. I'm just trying to rest and recover. I'm feeling considerably better, but still have a long way to go. Every day is a major struggle. There are so many things I want to do. It's been very frustrating lately. I should be getting progressively better, but there are more days than not that I actually feel worse. I'm doing everything right - eating healthy, exercising moderately, sleeping and resting.

On Monday, when the rest of the country was celebrating the red, white, and blue and going to the beach or having backyard BBQ's, I spent the day on the couch. I was beat. I started working on my book, and feel asleep in the middle of writing with the laptop on my lap. I realized as much as I had to declare war on cancer, I had to declare war on recovery.

I figured... it can't get any worse, right? I was bound and determined to do something... anything... to break my body of this fatigue. So I pushed it during one of my runs this week. Normally, I run to the Capitol and back. A short and slow jog sometimes sprinkled with a walk. As I reached the turn-around in front of the Capitol, as if right on cue...my cancer breakup song was the next song playing on my iPod. I had a choice. I could turn around and finish a short and slow run. Or I could run up Capitol Hill. I cranked up the volume so I wouldn't hear myself breathing hard... and I ran. The whole way up Capitol Hill. For those of you who have never seen Capitol Hill... it's a crazy steep hill. I ran to the top. The whole way. In my head... at the top was like the scene from Rocky where he climbed the steps in front of the museum and was jumping up and down. In reality, I had my head between my knees trying not to vomit on the grounds of our nation's Capitol. I caught my breath, and ran back to work with a pace I haven't seen in a long time.

I don't feel any better. But I don't feel worse. B12 is my new best friend.
Love, hugs, and breaking on through to the other side.

Holly

SPF AND A BIG FLOPPY HAT
July 17, 2011

The beach. Two outdoor concerts. Kings Dominion.

The question is.... What are the fun activities Holly has had to graciously decline this summer?

Thank you for your continued prayers, emails, thoughts, cards, and invitations between my recovery and Carter's deployment to Afghanistan. All are very much appreciated. Carter is putting in long hours but doing well and I hear from him several times a week. Please continue to keep his safety in your prayers.

My strength and energy have been coming back slowly. I can see progress, albeit small, from even a couple weeks ago. I don't know if it's pushing myself with the "more strenuous" workouts, the vitamins, lots of prayers, or just good old fashioned time, but I'll take it. I'm still waking up tired. But it's tired with energy.

While I've had to tone down participating in the bigger fun activities, I've been enjoying the small everyday gifts. Not having to take a nap (every day), taking Stepson out for ice cream, working on my book, and cleaning the house (yes I'm crazy I called cleaning the house a gift). I'm also walking to the pool, swimming laps, and then sitting under the umbrella with my favorite magazines and getting my quiet time on. Last count was 12 laps, and my end of summer goal is 20. For a former XTerra triathlete and someone who was able to swim two miles without blinking an eye, 20 laps is humbling, but will be a huge accomplishment.

Love, hugs, and not throwing in the towel, just grabbing one to walk to the pool. Holly

40 IS THE NEW 50
July 25, 2011

Being female, it is in my DNA to obsess over certain things, especially my weight and how my body looks. Add a sprinkle of cancer and cancer treatment to that equation and despite being ecstatically happy that I'm healthy, I am still dealing with a daily dose of, "I want my body back," "I want my energy back," and "I want my life back." My diet is clean and I'm faithful to the gym, so understandably frustrated when progress is going backwards instead of forwards.

I went to the medical professionals for their opinion. According to the oncology counselor, a few extra pounds is totally normal and a side effect of the cancer and treatment. Ohhhhh those are fighting words. And then some sage advice from the radiation oncologist, "40 is the new 50. Welcome to chemical menopause and all of its fun side effects." I-de-clare-war.

After being exhausted and down for the count all weekend, I woke up today feeling somewhat refreshed. So I ran. At 6:00 in the morning it was 85 degrees and 100% humidity so I was only wearing a sports bra and running shorts. Oh and the lymphodema sleeve which is so much fun to wear in this heat. (BTW...I. HATE. THAT. F*$#*!G. THING). And I got a "woo hoo" from some guy in a truck. Seriously dude? If anyone is looking for the President of the Jiggly-Muffin-Top-Lymphodema-Sleeve-Wearing-Fetish-Fan-Club... he's driving down Pennsylvania Avenue.

And then I arrived at Capitol Hill. My daily Everest. I stopped. Put on a good song. Turned up the volume. And it was an all-out assault to the top. Yes, I sprinted to the top of Capitol Hill. In this heat. I'm realizing this hill represents everything I'm hating on right now... the cancer... the recovery... my husband being away... stressful job... and the jiggly muffin top. After almost puking, and for a brief moment in time... all is well in my world.

Love, hugs, and making mole hills out of mountains.

Holly

SCAR TISSUE THAT I WISH YOU SAW
August 1, 2011

I'm holding a coupon for $1.00 off Scarzone. I'm not brand loyal, and I'm not an EXTREME couponer, but I do try to live frugally and will take a dollar off coupon to pay for the scar reducing cream, whatever brand it may be. The top scar is barely noticeable now. The bottom and bigger scar is still pretty big but it is healing and looking much better. Which is parallel to the scars inside. Still sizable, but healing and looking better.

I had been waiting. And I wasn't sure for what. But Saturday night at 8:00, which is normally the time my eyes are closing and I'm falling asleep, I was hit with some inspiration. I poured two ounces of wine and broke off a small piece of dark chocolate (yes, a wild and crazy Saturday night while my husband is deployed) and grabbed my laptop and started laying out a game plan. And I cranked for 30 minutes. I am determined to make something good come out of all of this. It's still swirling around in my head, so I'm not sharing any details yet. I might be paying $1.00 less for scar cream, but the healing inside is worth so much more. I know good things are yet to come... please say a prayer for this concept.

Love, hugs, and a young Virginia girl in a push-up bra,
Holly

BLIND FAITH
August 2, 2011

This morning, I'm standing on the corner in downtown DC, waiting to cross the street. A blind man approaches with his cane. Without the beeping crosswalks, how do you know when it's safe to cross the street? I closed my eyes to experience his world. Not only could you hear the shift in traffic, but you could actually feel the energy of the street change.

You don't need sight to have vision.

Today was just an average, ordinary, normal Tuesday. With two big exceptions.

I have been very blessed and have worked very hard to have a successful career. Cancer is a game changer. I inherited a family while going through this. It's not just me anymore. I have my health to take care of. And my boys to take care of. Last year, at the same time as this cancer thing started, I got a big promotion at work. But a demanding and stressful management job is not the best thing for me right now. After many months of deliberation, I decided to step down, and I signed the paperwork this morning. It was an extreme honor to be appointed to a very coveted position. It's a greater honor to have the support to shift my primary focus to my health and my boys.

That was my morning. My afternoon was three hours spent at the hospital going through the first round of post-treatment tests. Oh you know... the ones that determine if the cancer is gone. No big deal. The irony is that work has been so crazy lately, I didn't even have time to think about today's tests to the point where I actually forgot about them. Which is probably good. While Dr. S. has to give her official blessing next week, the techs reviewed all of the films and gave an initial declaration... HOLLY BERTONE IS CANCER FREE. (put your hands in the air shake your derriere).

Irony of ironies... August 2, 2010, I was at my first doctors appointment two days after finding the lump. Life always has a way of coming back around full circle.

Love, hugs, closing my eyes, and safely crossing the street.

Holly

MAKE A WISH
August 17, 2011

I was diagnosed with breast cancer on August 17, 2010. For years to come, today will be a celebration of survivorship. As I enter into middle age, this is something much better to look forward to than wrinkles.

Love, hugs, and blowing out one candle.

Holly

EPILOGUE

Dearest Warrior Sisters,

You are not alone and I hope this book brought you some smiles and inspiration. If you ever want to chat, please contact me. I would love to hear from you.

holly@coconutheadsurvivalguide.com

Love and hugs,

Holly

ABOUT THE AUTHOR

Holly Bertone is an author, blogger, and breast cancer survivor and advocate. She is the President and CEO of Pink Fortitude, LLC and Editor in Chief at the inspirational blog The Coconut Head's Survival Guide. Holly holds a Masters Degree from Johns Hopkins University, a Bachelor's Degree from Elizabethtown College, and is a Project Management Professional (PMP).

Holly is an Ambassador for the Tigerlily Foundation, was accepted into the National Cancer Survivor's Day Speaker Bureau, and was named a 2014 Woman of the Year by the National Association of Professional Women. She is passionate about reaching out to breast cancer survivors, and also volunteers for organizations supporting our military veterans. In her free time, she loves to garden, hit flea markets antique stores, and yard sales, and drink a cup of coffee on her back porch. Holly is married to a retired Green Beret, is a stepmother, and lives in Alexandria, VA.

You can follow and reach Holly:
Blog: http://coconutheadsurvivalguide.com
Social Media: @PinkFortitude
Email: holly@coconutheadsurvivalguide.com.

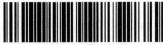

Made in the USA
San Bernardino, CA
07 June 2017